LONG-TERM CARE
FOR THE ELDERLY

LONG-TERM CARE FOR THE ELDERLY
A Factbook

David L. Rabin
Patricia Stockton

Funded by a Grant from the Robert Wood Johnson Foundation

New York   Oxford
OXFORD UNIVERSITY PRESS
1987

Oxford University Press

Oxford   New York   Toronto
Delhi   Bombay   Calcutta   Madras   Karachi
Petaling Jaya   Singapore   Hong Kong   Tokyo
Nairobi   Dar es Salaam   Cape Town
Melbourne   Auckland

and associated companies in

Beirut   Berlin   Ibadan   Nicosia

Copyright © 1987 by Oxford University Press, Inc.

Published by Oxford University Press, Inc.,
200 Madison Avenue, New York, New York 10016

Oxford is a registered trademark of Oxford University Press

Library of Congress Cataloging-in-Publication Data

Rabin, David.
  Long-term care for the elderly.

  "Funded by a grant from the Robert Wood Johnson Foundation."
  Includes bibliographies and index.
  1. Aged—Long term care—United States—Handbooks,
manuals, etc.   2. Aged—United States—Handbooks,
manuals, etc.   I. Stockton, Patricia, 1938–   .
II. Robert Wood Johnson Foundation.   III. Title.
[DNLM: 1. Health Services for the Aged—United
States.   2. Long Term Care—in old age. WT 30 R116L]
RA564.8R33   1987   362.1′9897′00973   86-23891
ISBN 0-19-504102-X

ISBN 0-19-504106-2 (pbk.)
9 8 7 6 5 4 3 2 1

9 8 7 6 5 4 3 2 1

Printed in the United States of America
on acid-free paper

Introduction

Long-term care encompasses a spectrum of medical, personal, and social services provided to aged and disabled individuals because of diminished capacity for self-care. Recent demographic, social, and economic changes have made long-term care a major issue in the field of health and social policy.

During the 1960's, health policy concerns were focused on ensuring equal access to medical care while maintaining the incomes of those aged 65 and over. Medicare, based on the insurance principle with fee-for-service reimbursements to providers, gave substantial protection to beneficiaries against the rising costs of hospital and some other acute health care services, while Medicaid provided additional assistance for those in greatest need.

From the time that these programs were introduced, expenditures far exceeded original projections due to a number of factors, including continuing high-cost technological innovation in the hospital sector, inflationary pressures within the economy as a whole, increases in the number of beneficiaries and in health care utilization, and demographic changes within the elderly population.

As a result, the debate in the 1980's is focused on the financing and provision of long-term care for an increasingly aged population in the context of economic constraints on all public expenditures, with particular pressure on the Medicare and Medicaid programs.

Since the early 1970's, there has been a major decline in mortality rates for all older age groups, including the most aged, with a consequent increase in life expectancy. The 1980 Census of the Population showed a higher proportion than had been previously projected of individuals aged 85, 95, and even 100 years and over. The elderly are now predicted to continue to increase as a proportion of the total population, with the highest rate of growth being among those aged 85 and over.

Until recently, little was known about the characteristics of the very old, since relatively few individuals aged 75 or 85 and over were included in surveys, and data were therefore aggregated for the total elderly population. It has now been shown that with advancing age there are substantial increases in morbidity, functional disability, and utilization rates for all health services, including acute hospital, nursing home, and home health care. Studies also show that at the present time the family is the major provider of care and assistance to the noninstitutionalized, functionally disabled elderly.

Publicly financed long-term care is largely institutional based, most care being provided in privately operated nursing homes reimbursed under the Medicaid program. Individuals who would not be eligible for Medicaid while living in the community may become eligible after admission to a nursing home by depleting their resources and "spending down" to eligibility levels.

In 1977 over 20 percent of all individuals aged 85 and over resided in nursing homes, and nursing home reimbursements account for the highest proportion of total Medicaid expenditures. While public expenditures for nursing home care increased constantly during the 1970's, a number of reports exposed the poor conditions that prevailed in many nursing homes and argued that institutional care was inappropriate for many of the nursing home population. The realization that continuing expansion of the nursing home sector to accommodate the same proportion of elderly individuals in the future is neither economically feasible nor socially desirable led to a search for alternatives in the provision of long-term care, with an emphasis on home- and community-based services.

Home health care benefits, restricted in range and coverage, have always been available to eligible Medicare and Medicaid recipients and, although the Medicare benefit was recently liberalized, the emphasis remains on care related to acute episodes of illness. A recent major change in reimbursement methods for hospital admissions under Medicare has produced strong incentives for earlier discharge of patients, with increased demand for posthospital nursing home or home health care. This change, together with extended home health benefits, has led to an increase in high-technology home care, in the number of home health agencies, particularly proprietary and hospital based, and in the proportion of the Medicare budget expended on home care. It is not clear that these changes benefit the high proportion of dependent elderly persons with long-term home management and personal care needs.

At the same time there have been legislative changes in the Medicaid program to encourage the development of home- and community-based services for individuals who would otherwise be institutionalized. Home- and community-based care is also funded under other federal programs such as the Older Americans Act, with additional funding from state and voluntary sources. There is considerable administrative fragmentation in the provision of these services, and little is known about the providers, the clients, or the adequacy of service provision to meet the growing needs of the aging population.

Many factors may have an impact on the need for and provision of care to the elderly, both now and in the future, including modifications to existing Medicare, Medicaid, and other federal programs; increasing labor force participation by women, the traditional care givers to the aged; and changes in the family structure and future income of the elderly. Although life expectancy has increased for both sexes, it is substantially higher for women than men, so that most very elderly women are widowed. Furthermore, income declines with age, so that in the absence of adequate financial assets the very elderly are unable to pay for needed assistance where family support or publicly funded programs are not available.

Demographic, social, and economic trends combined with frequent legislative and regulatory changes in the funding and provision of health and other social services mean that understanding the issues relating to long-term care is complex and supporting data are not readily available. Data relevant to long-term care are collected by many different agencies, including the Bureau of the Census, the National Center for Health Statistics, and the Health Care Financing Administration, both on a routine basis and from periodic surveys, but there is no comprehensive source for comparing data disseminated by different federal agencies. Furthermore, recent budget constraints have restricted the availability of published data from these agencies.

This book is therefore designed to serve as a concise reference source in areas where national data are available relating to long-term care for the elderly. It provides basic information on issues and legislation together with summary statistics of published and unpublished data obtained from different federal agencies. As far as possible, national trend data are presented to show how changes have occurred over time and are projected to continue in the future. We have also gathered data on differences by state, age, sex, and race that demonstrate variations within the elderly population. These data from national censuses and surveys have been supplemented by some relevant data from local studies. Each chapter is referenced for additional reading and data sources. Topic areas include population growth and change, mortality, morbidity, and functional disability, changes in family structure and living arrangements, in income, and in dependency ratios between the elderly and younger generations. Chapters on health care expenditures and utilization and on growth and change in the nursing home sector are also included. In view of the recent shift in policy from institutional to community-based care, home health and related care has been treated in three separate chapters on the home care population, home health provision under Medicare and Medicaid, and services provided under other federal programs. There is also a brief review of some of the research and initiatives being undertaken with regard to long-term care for the elderly. Finally, there is a section on international comparisons to demonstrate that population aging is not unique to the United States and that all industrialized countries have the same concerns in providing long-term care to an increasing proportion of elderly persons.

Although there is evidence that there are as many severely impaired

individuals in the younger population as among the elderly, the rate of
growth of the elderly population presents a unique problem in the provision and planning of services and in the allocation of resources.
Changes are constantly occurring in the funding and provision of care in
both the public and private sectors. It is too soon to assess the impact of
some recent developments, while for others national data are not available: improved access for Medicare enrollees to more comprehensive prepaid health care in health maintenance organizations; the development
of "life care communities" and specialized housing for the elderly; and
the promotion of long-term care insurance by the private insurance market. Acknowledging the limitations of the data presented, we hope this
book will serve as a basic reference source for all those with a personal or
professional interest in understanding the dimensions of the problems
associated with the aging of the population and in planning and implementing appropriate programs.

Washington, D.C.   D.L.R.
January 1986   P.S.

Acknowledgments

When the idea of developing a reference source for data relating to the complexities of the provision of long-term care for the elderly was first conceived, it was discussed with Bruce Vladeck, who gave active encouragement and advice for pursuing the idea.

Many thanks go to Jeffrey Merrill who offered help and support in the planning stages; while he was director of the Center for Health Policy Studies at Georgetown University, he served on the advisory committee for the book and continued his support after his move to the Robert Wood Johnson Foundation.

Acknowledgments and appreciation are given to the other members of the advisory committee for their help in advising on the contents and, subsequently, in reviewing and revising the various sections of the book. These members were: Charles Fisher of the Health Care Financing Administration, Jacob Feldman of the National Center for Health Statistics, Karen Rak of Home Health Line, George Greenberg of the Office of the Assistant Secretary for Planning and Evaluation, and Jacob Siegel of the Center for Population Research at Georgetown University and the Bureau of the Census. We also thank all the other individuals, too numerous to mention, in the Health Care Financing Administration, the National Center for Health Statistics, and other agencies for assisting with the provision of information and data.

Most important, we thank the Robert Wood Johnson Foundation for funding the proposal, thus enabling us to make the concept a reality.

Gratitude also goes to Roger Plaskett for his constant support and encouragement, to Andy Lohmeier for entering the data, and to Alan Zuckerman for his technical advice and for writing the program which facilitated the preparation of the tables for publication.

Contents

1. Demography, 3
2. Family Structure and Living Arrangements, 19
3. Income of the Elderly, 34
4. Mortality, Morbidity, and Functional Disability, 52
5. Health Care Expenditures and Utilization, 79
6. Nursing Homes, 113
7. Home Care: The Population and the System, 140
8. Home Health Care: The Reimbursement System, 159
9. Community and Social Support Services, 184
10. The Veterans Administration, 204
11. Research, Demonstrations, and Initiatives in Long-Term Care, 215
12. International Comparisons of Population Aging and Long-Term Care Financing and Provision, 226

Index, 243

Tables

1-1. Actual and projected growth of the total population of the United States, and the population aged 65 and over, 1900–2050. 6

1-2. Life expectancy at birth and at age 65, by race and sex, selected years 1900–1983. 7

1-3. Life expectancy at birth and at age 65 by sex, selected years 1900 to 1980, with projections to 2050. 8

1-4. Actual percentage of the total population in older age groups, 1960 and 1980, with projections from 1990 to 2020. 9

1-5. Percentage distribution of the population 65 and over by age group, 1960 and 1980, with projections from 1990 to 2020. 9

1-6. Projected growth of the total white population and the white population aged 55 and over, 1990 to 2050. 10

1-7. Projected growth of the total black population and the black population aged 55 and over, 1990 to 2050. 11

1-8. Projected growth of the total female population and the female population aged 55 and over, 1990 to 2050. 12

1-9. Projected growth of the total male population and the male population aged 55 and over, 1990 to 2050. 13

1-10. Projections of the population aged 85 and over, 1990 to 2050. 14

1-11. Total population and rank by state, population aged 65 and over and rank by state, elderly as a percentage of the total population, 1980, and percentage increase in the elderly, 1970–1980. 15

1-12. Estimated net migration of the population cohort aged 65 and over at mid-decade, by state, 1970–1980 and 1960–1970. 16

1-13. Population aged 65 and over and 85 and over, and percentage of the total elderly population aged 85 and over, by state, 1981. 17

2-1. Familial aged dependency ratios, with one elderly generation and with two elderly generations, actual and projected series, 1930–2030. 22

2-2. Distribution of the male population aged 55 years and over, by marital status and by age, 1960 to 1981 with projections to 1995. 23

2-3. Distribution of the female population aged 55 years and over, by marital status and by age, 1960 to 1981 with projections to 1995.   24

2-4. Marital status of the total white population and the white population aged 55 and over, 1981.   25

2-5. Marital status of the total black population and the black population aged 55 and over, 1981.   26

2-6. Divorced persons per 1,000 married persons with spouse present, by age, sex and race, 1960, 1970, 1980 and 1983.   27

2-7. Living arrangements of the elderly, 1970 and 1983.   29

2-8. Living arrangements of the male population aged 65 and over, and living arrangements of the female population aged 65 and over, 1965, 1975 and 1981.   30

2-9. Number and percentage of the total population aged 65 and over in long-term institutions, 1950, 1960, 1970, and 1980.   31

3-1. Percentage distribution of money income from particular sources for aged units 55 and over, 1980 and 1982.   38

3-2. Median income of aged units by age, sex and marital status, 1980 and 1982.   40

3-3. Income distribution of the total white and black populations and of those aged 55 and over, 1979.   41

3-4. Income distribution of the total male and female populations and of those aged 55 and over, 1979.   42

3-5. Median income for households with the householder aged 65 or over, by race and by state, 1979.   43

3-6. Poverty rates for selected elderly subgroups, 1982.   44

3-7. Maximum potential dollar value of Supplemental Security Income and food stamp benefits for aged individuals by state, January 1984.   45

3-8. Labor force participation ratios for the population 55 years and over, by age, race and sex, selected years 1955–1981.   46

3-9. Social Security population and dependency ratios by broad age group, 1960–2060.   47

3-10. Comparison of OASDI beneficiaries and covered workers, 1945–2060.   49

4-1. Death rates of the population aged 65 and over, by age group, and percentage change over time, 1950, 1960, 1970, 1980 and 1983.   56

4-2. Age-specific and age-adjusted death rates for 10 leading causes, 1979, 1981 and 1982.   57

4-3. Ratio of male to female death rates for the ten leading causes of death for the population 65 years and over, by age, 1978. 58

4-4. Deaths and death rates per 100,000 population in specified group, by age, race and sex, 1982. 60–61

4-5. Ratio of black and other races to white death rates for the ten leading causes of death for the population 65 years and over, by age, 1978. 62

4-6. Number of persons affected and morbidity rates of the fifteen most prevalent chronic conditions for the total population and those aged 65 and over, 1981. 63

4-7. Prevalence rates of leading chronic conditions in noninstitutionalized persons aged 65 and over, by sex, 1979. 64

4-8. Prevalence rates of senility per 1,000 nursing home residents, by age and sex, 1977. 65

4-9. Illustration of the effect of population changes in the U.S. between 1980 and 2005 on selected indices of mental disorders, assuming 1980 rates applied to the projected population, by race, for 2005. 67

4-10. Rates of need for assistance in the noninstitutionalized elderly population, by type of need and by age, 1979. 68

4-11. Number and percentage distribution of the total Medicare population and of functionally impaired elderly, living in the community, by age, race and sex, 1982. 70

4-12. Percentage distribution of the number of IADL limitations reported by functionally disabled elderly living in the community, by age, race and sex, 1982. 71

4-13. Percentage distribution of functionally disabled elderly, living in the community, by type of IADL limitation, and by age, race and sex, 1982. 72

4-14. Percentage distribution of number of ADL limitations reported by functionally disabled elderly living in the community, and by age, race and sex, 1982. 73

4-15. Percentage distribution of functionally disabled elderly, living in the community, reporting ADL limitations, by type of activity, and by age, race and sex, 1982. 74

4-16. Probability of change in functional status between years 1.25 and 6, by initial functional state and age for elderly persons living in the community: Massachusetts, 1974–1980. 75

5-1. Aggregate and per capita national health expenditures by source of funds and as a percentage of gross national product, selected years 1929–1983. 84–85

5-2. Percentage distribution of personal health care expenditures by source of funds, selected years 1929–1983. 86

5-3. Average annual growth in personal health expenditures, total population growth, growth of population aged 65 and over, and effect of aging on health expenditures, by state, 1966–1978. 88

5-4. Aggregate health care expenditures and percentage distribution for the population aged 65 and over, by type of expenditure and source of funds, selected years, 1965 to 1984. 90–91

5-5. Total per capita personal health care expenditures and percentage distribution for individuals aged 65 and over, by source of funds and type of service, 1984. 92

5-6. Medicare expenditures and percentage distribution by type of service, selected years 1967–1983. 93

5-7. Medicare utilization: number of aged beneficiaries enrolled and served and percentage change, by type of service, 1967, 1980, 1981, and 1982. 94

5-8. Medicare utilization: amount reimbursed for aged beneficiaries and percentage change by type of service, 1967, 1980, 1981 and 1982. 95

5-9. Selected measures of use of Medicare benefits by decedents in their last year of life, and by survivors, according to age, in 1978. 96

5-10. Medicare reimbursement per enrollee and percentage distribution of total reimbursement for decedents in the last and second-to-last years of life, and for survivors, by type of service, in 1977 and 1978. 97

5-11. Medicaid expenditures and percentage distribution by type of service, selected years 1967–1983. 99

5-12. Unduplicated number of recipients under Medicaid by selected medical services, 1972–1983. 100–101

5-13. Medicaid vendor payments, by type of medical service, 1972–1983. 102–103

5-14. Medicaid recipients aged 65 and over as a percentage of total recipients, by state, 1975, 1977, 1979, 1981, 1983. 104

5-15. Personal health care expenditures for individuals aged 65 and over 1977, 1980, 1984, 1989. 107

5-16. Median out-of-pocket charges and mean percentage of charges and of family income that was made out-of-pocket, by selected characteristics, 1980. 108

5-17. Personal health care expenditures as a percentage of income for individuals aged 65 and over in 1977, 1980, 1984 and 1989. 109

6-1. Number of nursing homes and beds, percentage change and average bed size of homes, 1963, 1967, 1969, 1971, 1973, 1976, 1980 and 1982. 117

6-2. Number of persons 65 years and over, nursing and related care homes, beds, beds per 1,000 population aged 65 and over, and rank, by state, 1980. 118

6-3. Beds per 1,000 population aged 65 and over in nursing and related care homes with 25 or more beds, by state, selected years, 1969–1980. 120

6-4. Number and percentage distribution of nursing and related care homes with 25 or more beds, by bed size and type of ownership, selected years 1969–1980. 121

6-5. Full-time equivalent employees per 100 beds in nursing and related care homes with 25 or more beds, by bed size and type of ownership, selected years 1969–1980. 122

6-6. Number and percentage distribution of nursing home residents by age, 1977. 122

6-7. Comparison of nursing home resident population and the general population, by age, 1977. 123

6-8. Number of nursing home residents and percentage distribution by primary source of payment and by sex, age, marital status and race, 1977. 124–125

6-9. Number and percentage distribution of nursing home residents by index of dependency in activities of daily living, by selected resident characteristics, 1977. 126–127

6-10. Total beds in certified facilities, beds per 1,000 population, beds per 1,000 population aged 65 and over and beds per 1,000 population aged 85 and over, by state, 1981. 129

6-11. Total beds in certified facilities, percentage certified for Medicare and Medicaid, and percentage certified for Medicaid only, by state, 1981. 130

6-12. Medicare certified skilled nursing facility beds and Medicare reimbursed days per 1,000 persons aged 65 and over, by state, 1979. 131

6-13. Percentage of all Medicaid recipients in skilled and intermediate care facilities, by state, 1983. 133

6-14. Calendar year estimates of expenditures for nursing home care, in millions of dollars, by source of payment and as a percentage of total payments, selected years, 1965–1983. 134

6-15. Total Medicaid expenditures, by state, and percentage of total expenditures for skilled and intermediate care, 1983. 135

6-16. Distribution of nursing home residents by age in 1977, and projections of the number in selected years, based on 1977 utilization rates.   136

7-1. Assistance needed by functionally disabled elderly living in the community to perform specified activities of daily living, by age, 1982.   144–145

7-2. Percentage distribution of the total population aged 65 and over, and the home care population aged 65 and over, by selected characteristics, 1979.   146

7-3. Need for home care for selected population characteristics, by age: prevalence rate per 1,000 persons aged 65 and over, 1979.   148

7-4. Percentage of the elderly needing personal care assistance and percentage needing home management assistance, by living arrangement, age and sex, 1979 and 1980.   149

7-5. Percentage distribution of sources of home care assistance for elderly persons living in the community, by type of need for those living with a spouse and those living with other relatives, 1979.   150

7-6. Percentage distribution of functionally disabled elderly living in the community, by ADL level and by source of assistance, 1982.   151

7-7. Distribution of hours per week of informal care provided to noninstitutionalized, disabled elderly, by source of care, sex and marital status, 1982.   153

7-8. Sources of payment for home care reported by functionally disabled elderly persons living in the community, receiving paid home care, unadjusted and adjusted for unknown response, 1982. 154

7-9. Characteristics of all disabled elderly and of those paying privately for home care, 1982.   155

8-1. Total Medicare reimbursements, reimbursements for home health services, number of home health visits and percentage change, 1969–1983.   164

8-2. Medicare utilization of home health services, selected calendar years, 1975–1983.   165

8-3. Medicare: percentage distribution of persons served, by number of home health visits, selected calendar years, 1975, 1980 and 1982.   166

8-4. Medicare: home health agency charges, average charge per visit and percentage change, by census region and division, 1981 and 1983.   167

8-5. Medicare: home health agency charges, average charge per visit and percentage change, by state, 1981 and 1983.   168

8-6. Medicare: all home health visits, nursing visits and percentage change, by census region and division, 1981 and 1983.   169

8-7. Medicare: all home health visits, nursing visits and percentage change, by state, 1981 and 1983.   170

8-8. Revenue sources of Medicare-certified home health agencies, 1982.   171

8-9. Distribution of Medicare-certified home health agencies, by auspices, and percentage change over time, 1972, 1982 and 1985.   172

8-10. Medicare: percentage distribution of persons receiving home health visits, and charges, by type of agency, 1975, 1980 and 1982.   174–175

8-11. Number of home health agencies providing in-home services, by type of service and by staff or other arrangements, January 1984.   176

8-12. Distribution of persons served by type of home health service, selected years, 1974–1980.   176

8-13. Average number of full-time equivalent staff employed by home health agencies, by staff skill level and by auspices, January 1982.

8-14. Medicare home health services for the elderly: persons served and visits, by age, 1977 and 1980.   178

8-15. Medicaid home health services: payments and recipients and percentage change, 1972–1983.   179

8-16. Medicaid: total payments and medical vendor payments for home health services, and as a percentage of total Medicaid payments, by state, 1983.   180

8-17. Medicaid: total recipients, home health recipients and home health recipients as a percentage of the total, by state, 1983.   182

9-1. Title XX, Social Services Block Grant: services to be provided by states, 1984.   186

9-2. Title XX, Social Services Block Grant: distribution of proposed services that may benefit the elderly, by state, 1984.   188–189

9-3. Older Americans Act: Title 111 expenditures by service category and percentage distribution, fiscal years 1981 and 1982.   192

9-4. National Data Base on Aging: Area Agency on Aging service expenditures, 1982 and 1983.   193

9-5. Area Agency on Aging: number of clients and percentage distribution by age and service category, October 1, 1983–September 30, 1984.   194

9-6. Area Agency on Aging: number of clients and percentage distribution by sex and service category, October 1, 1983–September 30, 1984. 195

9-7. Area Agency on Aging: number of clients and percentage distribution by marital status and service category, October 1, 1983–September 30, 1984. 196

9-8. Area Agency on Aging: number of clients and percentage distribution by living arrangement and service category, October 1, 1983–September 30, 1984. 197

9-9. Medicaid noninstitutional long-term care: states providing personal care and adult day care, 1981. 199

9-10. Federal and state expenditures on optional state supplements to recipients living in non-medical long-term care facilities, for states with federally-administered Supplemental Security Income programs, 1982. 201

10-1. Veterans population by age cohort, selected years, 1980–2030. 209

10-2. Veterans Administration: inpatient care summary, 1982. 210

10-3. Percentage use of Veterans Administration institutional care, by age, 1982. 211

10-4. Use of Veterans Administration hospital and nursing home care by aged veterans, 1982. 212

11-1. Summary of changes to the Medicaid program under 2176 Waivers for Home and Community-Based Care. 222

11-2. Medicaid 2176 Waivers for Home and Community-Based Care: number of states, by service offered and eligibility group, April 1985. 223

11-3. Medicaid 2176 Waivers for Home and Community-Based Care: number of approved waivers, by service offered, April 1985. 224

12-1. Estimates of the percentage of the population aged 65 and over, 75 and over, and 80 and over, selected countries, 1980 and 2000. 232

12-2. Life expectancy at birth, by sex, selected countries. 233

12-3. Life expectancy at ages 65, 75 and 85, by sex, selected countries, 1980–82. 233

12-4. Total health expenditures as a percentage of gross national product, public health expenditures as a percentage of gross domestic product, and percentage change 1960–1980, selected countries. 235

12-5. Total public expenditures on the elderly and as a percentage of gross national product, and total public health expenditures on the elderly, and as a percentage of gross national product, selected countries.   237

12-6. Population aged 65 and over in institutions and group living quarters as a percentage of the total population aged 65 and over, selected countries.   239

LONG-TERM CARE
FOR THE ELDERLY

1

Demography

Census data show that between 1900 and 1980 the total population of the United States increased by nearly 200 percent, from just over 76 million to 226.5 million. During this period, the population aged 65 and over increased over 700 percent, from a little over 3 million to 25.5 million. Whereas in 1900 those aged 65 and over represented only 4 percent of the population, by 1980 the proportion had grown to 11.3 percent. The number of individuals aged 65 and over doubled between 1950 and 1980.

Within the elderly population, the sector showing the greatest growth in recent decades is comprised of those aged 85 and over. Their numbers increased by nearly 1700 percent, from 123,000 to 2.2 million, or from 0.16 to 1.0 percent of the total population, between 1900 and 1980, and it is predicted that by 2020 there will be 7 million individuals in this age group, representing 2.5 percent of the total population.

Changes in the absolute numbers of individuals in the various age groups of the total population and changes in the age structure, or relative size of these age groups, are a function of mortality, fertility, and migration. The U.S. Bureau of the Census has developed "highest-," "lowest-," and "middle-" series projections of the future population, based on alternative assumptions of fertility, mortality, and net immigration. The middle-range assumptions represent the likely future course of population growth; high- and low-range assumptions define a reasonable range of error.[1]

Middle-series projections of population growth to the middle of the next century assume the following: that fertility rates will stay constant at 1.9 lifetime births per woman; that life expectancy will increase slowly to 79.6 years by 2050, and that net immigration will remain constant at 450,000 per year. The highest and lowest projections of population growth are based on assumptions of life expectancy ranging between 83.3 and 76.7 years in 2050, with fertility rates from a high of 2.3 down to 1.6 lifetime births per woman, and net annual immigration from 750,000 to 250,000 persons.

Fertility

Rapid increases in the number of births occurring in a predominantly young population in the early part of the 20th century, combined with declining infant mortality, largely account for the current increase in absolute numbers of the elderly population. During the 1920's and 1930's, fertility rates were low, but the twenty years following the end of World War II in 1945 are described as the "baby boom" years because of the very high birthrates. Fertility patterns have changed again during the twenty years from 1965 to 1985, birthrates having declined and remained constant in recent years. Projections are based on recent fertility patterns, women's expectations of future births, and social and economic trends to lower fertility, such as an increase in labor force participation, higher educational attainment, and age at first marriage.[2]

It is the aging of the "baby boom" cohorts, who will begin to reach age 65 in about the year 2010, combined with projections of low to moderate future fertility rates, that leads to the confident prediction of a major increase in the elderly population, both in absolute numbers and as a percentage of the total population.

Mortality

A decline in fertility rates always contributes to a rise in the proportion of the older population, and vice versa. A decrease in mortality rates will lead to an increase in the proportion of elderly only if the changes are concentrated in the older population.[1] The accuracy of projections of the number of Americans in each older age group depends on the accuracy of mortality assumptions. In the past twenty-five years population projections have been too conservative with respect to mortality declines, particularly among the elderly; this accounts for a major proportion of the error in previous population forecasting.[1]

For the first half of this century death-rate declines were greater for the younger than the older population. During the past fifteen years, improvements have been greater for the elderly, including the very old, than for many younger age groups. Between 1960 and 1983 there was a 31-percent decline in mortality rates for those aged 75 to 84 and a 23-percent decline for those aged 85 and over. This major decrease in death rates has been responsible for changes within the age structure of the elderly population as an increasing number of individuals survive to advanced old age.

Modest continuing declines in mortality, with consequent increases in life expectancy, are projected to continue for all age groups. (For actual age, race, sex, and disease-specific mortality data and a discussion of future trends, see Chapter 4.)

Migration

Mass immigration of young Europeans before World War I had a major effect on population growth and on the number of individuals reaching age 65 prior to 1960. It is projected that in the future immigration will have a limited impact on the size and age structure of the total population.[1]

Assuming that there are no extraordinary movements of refugees, it is estimated that net migration will remain relatively constant at 450,000 per year into the next century. An immigration rate at or below this level would lead to zero population growth after the middle of the next century, if middle-range mortality and fertility assumptions are correct.[3]

Net immigration has, however, become a significant component of population projection error because of the recent high numbers of refugees and illegal immigrants. Population estimates now include estimates for these groups from data supplied by the Immigration and Naturalization Service.[3]

There is considerable population movement within the United States, and migration patterns of the elderly within and between states does affect the total distribution of the elderly population. This may become an increasingly important factor in the planning and provision of services for the elderly.

DATA SOURCES

Sources of information for the tables presented in this chapter are as follows.

The U.S. Bureau of the Census is the main source of demographic data in the United States, from the decennial census of the population and from periodic surveys published as Current Population Reports.[2,3] Other population estimates are provided by the Social Security Administration, using program enrollment data.

The National Center for Health Statistics maintains the National Vital Statistics System and collects data on births, marriages, divorces, and deaths through cooperative arrangements with state registration systems. These are used to develop statistics on mortality, life expectancy, and fertility rates.[4]

Population Growth and Life Expectancy

Table 1-1 shows the actual and projected growth of the total population of the United States and of the population aged 65 and over, from 1900 to 2050, together with the percentage of the elderly in the total population. It is predicted that the total population aged 65 and over will double in the fifty years from 1980 to 2030, and that the percentage aged 85 and over will increase in every decade until 2050.

As shown in Tables 1-2 and 1-3, life expectancy at birth has increased in nearly all time periods during this century, for all sex, race, and age

Table 1-1. Actual and projected growth of the total population of the United States and the population aged 65 and over, 1900-2050.

| Year | Total all ages | Age groups | | | |
		65 & over	65-74	75-84	85 & over
		Numbers in thousands			
1900	76,303	3,084	2,189	772	123
1910	91,972	3,950	2,793	989	167
1920	105,711	4,933	3,464	1,259	210
1930	122,775	6,634	4,721	1,641	272
1940	131,669	9,019	6,375	2,278	365
1950	150,697	12,270	8,415	3,278	577
1960	179,323	16,560	10,997	4,633	929
1970	203,302	19,980	12,447	6,124	1,409
1980	226,505	25,544	15,578	7,727	2,240
1990*	249,731	31,799	18,054	10,284	3,461
2000	267,955	35,036	17,677	12,318	4,926
2010	283,238	39,269	20,318	12,326	6,551
2020	296,597	51,386	29,855	14,486	7,081
2030	304,807	64,345	34,535	21,434	8,603
2040	308,559	66,643	29,272	24,882	12,834
2050	309,488	67,061	30,114	21,263	16,034
		Percentages			
1900	100.0	4.0	2.9	1.0	0.2
1910	100.0	4.3	3.0	1.1	0.2
1920	100.0	4.7	3.3	1.2	0.2
1930	100.0	5.4	3.8	1.3	0.2
1940	100.0	6.8	4.8	1.7	0.3
1950	100.0	8.1	5.6	2.2	0.4
1960	100.0	9.2	6.1	2.6	0.5
1970	100.0	9.8	6.1	3.0	0.7
1980	100.0	11.3	6.9	3.4	1.0
1990*	100.0	12.7	7.2	4.1	1.4
2000	100.0	13.1	6.6	4.6	1.9
2010	100.0	13.9	7.2	4.3	2.4
2020	100.0	17.3	10.0	4.8	2.5
2030	100.0	21.1	11.3	6.9	2.9
2040	100.0	21.6	9.5	8.0	4.2
2050	100.0	21.7	9.7	6.8	5.2

* Middle-series projections.

Source: U.S. Bureau of the Census, Decennial Censuses of Population 1900 to 1980, and U.S. Bureau of the Census, Current Population Reports, Series P-25, No. 952, Projections of the population of the United States by age, race and sex: 1983 to 2080. Washington, D.C., U.S. Government Government Printing Office, 1984

Table 1-2. Life expectancy at birth and at age 65, by race and sex, selected years 1900-1983.

	Total			Total		
Year	Both sexes	Male	Female	Both sexes	Male	Female
	At birth			At age 65		
1900*	47.3	46.3	48.3	11.9	11.5	12.2
1950	68.2	65.6	71.1	13.9	12.8	15.0
1960	69.7	66.6	73.1	14.3	12.8	15.8
1970	70.9	67.1	74.8	15.2	13.1	17.0
1975	72.6	68.8	76.6	16.1	13.8	18.1
1980	73.7	70.0	77.5	16.4	14.1	18.3
1982**	74.6	70.9	78.2	16.8	14.5	18.8
1983**	74.7	71.0	78.3	16.8	14.5	18.8

	White			White		
	Both sexes	Male	Female	Both sexes	Male	Female
Year	At birth			At age 65		
1900-1902*	47.6	46.6	48.7	---	11.5	12.2
1950	69.1	66.5	72.2	---	12.8	15.1
1960	70.6	67.4	74.1	14.4	12.9	15.9
1970	71.7	68.0	75.6	15.2	13.1	17.1
1975	73.4	69.5	77.3	16.1	13.8	18.2
1980	74.4	70.7	78.1	16.5	14.2	18.5
1982**	75.1	71.5	78.8	16.8	14.5	18.9
1983**	75.2	71.6	78.8	16.9	14.5	18.9

	Black			Black		
	Both sexes	Male	Female	Both sexes	Male	Female
Year	At birth			At age 65		
1900-1902*	33.0	32.5	33.5	---	10.4	11.4
1950	60.7	58.9	62.7	13.9	12.9	14.9
1960	63.2	60.7	65.9	13.9	12.7	15.1
1970	64.1	60.0	68.3	14.2	12.5	15.7
1975	66.8	62.4	71.3	15.0	13.1	16.7
1980	68.0	63.7	72.3	14.8	12.9	16.5
1982**	69.3	64.9	73.5	15.4	13.3	17.2
1983**	69.6	65.2	73.8	15.4	13.2	17.2

* Death registration area only. The death registration area increased from 10 states and the District of Columbia in 1900 to the coterminous United States in 1933.

** Provisional data.

Source: National Center for Health Statistics. Health, United States, 1984. DHHS Pub. No. (PHS)85-1232, Public Health Service. Washington, D.C. U.S. Government Printing Office, December 1984.

Table 1-3. Life expectancy at birth and at age 65 by sex, selected years 1900 to 1980, with projections to 2050.

	Male		Female	
Year	At birth	At age 65	At birth	At age 65
1900	46.56	11.35	49.07	12.01
1910	50.20	11.38	53.67	12.10
1920	54.59	11.81	56.33	12.34
1930	58.01	11.38	61.36	12.91
1940	60.89	11.92	65.34	13.42
1950	65.33	12.81	70.90	15.07
1960	66.58	12.91	73.19	15.89
1970	67.05	13.14	74.80	17.12
1980	69.85	14.02	77.53	18.35
1990*	72.29	15.11	79.85	19.92
2000	73.42	15.71	81.05	20.81
2010	73.93	15.08	81.62	21.27
2020	74.42	16.45	82.18	21.73
2030	74.90	16.81	82.74	22.18
2040	75.37	17.18	83.29	22.64
2050	75.84	17.55	83.84	23.11

* Middle-series projections.

Source: Aging America: trends and projections. Prepared by the Senate Special Committee on Aging in conjunction with the American Association of Retired Persons.

groups. A woman reaching age 65 in 1900 could expect to live 12 more years; by 1950 this had risen to 15 years. Life expectancy has recently increased at an accelerated rate, so that by 1980 it was 18.5 years for white women and 16.5 for black women at age 65. Although male life expectancy has not increased at the same rate, there is the same difference between black and white males as between black and white females. Table 1-3 indicates that life expectancy at birth and at age 65 is projected to increase steadily for both sexes into the middle of the next century, and the disparity between male and female life expectancy is expected to persist.

Table 1-4 shows the actual percentage of the total population at older age groups from 1960 to 1980 and projections from 1990 to 2020. The proportion aged 60 and over is projected to remain relatively stable from 1990 until 2010, while the proportions of older age groups—75, 80, and 85 and over—are projected to increase in each decade. The percentage of the population aged 60 and over will increase after 2010 with the aging of the baby boom cohorts. This change is reflected in Table 1-5, which shows the distribution of the population aged 65 and over between 1960 and 1980, with projections to 2020. The elderly population will continue to "age" until 2010, when the increase in the number of "young old" will change the percentage distributions.

Table 1-4. Actual percentage of the total population in older age groups, 1960 and 1980, with projections from 1990 to 2020*

			Year			
Age	1960	1980	1990	2000	2010	2020
60 & over	13.2	15.7	17.0	17.0	19.5	24.0
65 & over	9.3	11.3	12.7	13.1	13.9	17.3
70 & over	5.8	7.4	8.7	9.7	9.7	11.7
75 & over	3.1	4.4	5.5	6.5	6.7	7.3
80 & over	1.4	2.3	3.0	3.8	4.3	4.4
85 & over	0.5	1.0	1.4	1.9	2.4	2.5

* Middle-series projections.

Source: U.S. Bureau of the Census, Current Population Reports, Series P-23, No. 138, Demographic and socioeconomic aspects of aging in the United States. Washington, D.C., U.S. Government Printing Office, 1984.

Tables 1-6 and 1-7 show the projected growth of the total population and of population cohorts aged 55 and over, together with the percentage increase, for the white and the black populations between 1990 and 2050. The comparable projections for the male and female populations are shown in Tables 1-8 and 1-9. The overall growth rates for males and females are projected to be similar, but the older black population is projected to increase at two to three times the rate of the white population between 1990 and 2030. Also, while an actual decline in the white pop-

Table 1-5. Percentage distribution of the population 65 and over by age group, 1960 and 1980, with projections from 1990 to 2020*

			Year			
Age	1960	1980	1990	2000	2010	2020
65 & over	100.0	100.0	100.0	100.0	100.0	100.0
65 - 69	37.7	34.2	31.5	26.0	29.8	32.3
70 - 74	28.6	26.6	25.3	24.5	21.9	25.6
75 - 79	18.5	18.7	19.6	20.7	17.1	17.0
80 - 84	9.6	11.6	12.8	14.2	13.9	10.8
85 & over	5.6	8.8	10.9	14.7	17.4	14.3

* Middle-series projections.

Source: U.S. Bureau of the Census, Current Population Reports, Series P-23, No. 138, Demographic and socioeconomic aspects of aging in the United States. Washington, D.C., U.S. Government Printing Office, 1984.

Table 1-6. Projected growth of the total white population and the white population aged 55 and over, 1990 to 2050*

Year	White population (all ages)	Age groups			
		55–64	65–74	75–84	85 & over
		Numbers in thousands			
1990	210,790	18,536	16,226	9,352	3,019
2000	222,654	20,605	15,589	11,093	4,444
2010	231,654	29,769	17,635	10,863	5,680
2020	238,739	33,561	25,544	12,572	6,229
2030	241,647	27,565	28,814	18,329	7,456
2040	240,948	27,595	23,738	20,752	10,946
2050	238,314	29,283	23,942	17,230	13,371
		Percentage increase			
1990	-	-	-	-	-
2000	5.6	11.2	4.0	18.6	47.2
2010	4.0	44.5	13.0	-2.0	27.8
2020	3.1	12.7	44.8	15.7	9.7
2030	1.2	-18.0	17.4	45.8	19.7
2040	-0.3	0.0	-17.4	13.2	46.8
2050	-1.0	6.1	0.9	-17.0	22.2

* Middle-series projections.

Source: U.S. Bureau of the Census, Current Population Reports, Series P-25, No. 952, Projections of the population of the United States, by age, race and sex: 1983 to 2080. Washington, D.C., U.S. Government Printing Office, 1984.

ulation aged 55 and over is predicted after 2040, the black population 55 and over is projected to show continued growth, but at a slower rate.

The effects of the aging of the "baby boom" cohorts are graphically illustrated in these tables, with 45-percent increases in the number in age groups in successive decades for the white population and for males and females after 2010 and even greater increases in successive age groups for the black population.

Table 1-10 shows projections for the total population aged 85 and over and the percentage distribution of those aged 85 to 89, 90 to 94, 95 to 99 and 100 years and over, from 1990 to 2050. Some variation in the percentage distributions with successive decades is predicted, and although it is suggested that even the population of those aged 100 years and over will continue to grow, the evidence for this constant major increase in survival rates for the very aged is disputed.[5]

Distribution of the Older Population

Table 1-11 shows, by state, the distribution of the total population, the number and percentage of those aged 65 and over, and the percentage

Table 1-7. Projected growth of the total black population and the black population aged 55 and over, 1990 to 2050*

Year	Black population (all ages)	Age groups			
		55-64	65-74	75-84	85 & over
		Numbers in thousands			
1990	31,412	1,998	1,475	847	257
2000	35,753	2,355	1,589	975	412
2010	40,033	3,747	1,928	1,090	541
2020	44,175	5,115	3,104	1,355	645
2030	47,598	4,716	4,262	2,412	831
2040	50,329	5,158	3,964	3,050	1,355
2050	52,297	5,936	4,404	2,859	1,964
		Percentage increase			
1990	-	-	-	-	-
2000	14.0	17.9	7.7	15.1	60.1
2010	12.0	59.1	21.3	11.8	31.3
2020	10.3	36.5	61.0	24.3	19.2
2030	7.7	-8.0	37.0	78.0	28.8
2040	5.7	9.4	-7.0	26.5	63.0
2050	3.9	15.0	11.0	-6.0	45.0

* Middle-series projections.

Source: U.S. Bureau of the Census, Current Population Reports, Series P-25, No. 952, Projections of the population of the United States by age, race and sex: 1983 to 2080. Washington, D.C., U.S. Government Printing Office, 1984.

increase from 1970 to 1980. Florida has the highest proportion of population aged 65 and over, and it experienced an increase of over 71 percent in the size of this population group from 1970 to 1980. Other states in the South and West with relatively small populations, such as Nevada, Arizona, and New Mexico, also experienced major increases in the population aged 65 and over. A major factor contributing to the growth of the elderly in most of these "Sunbelt" states is migration from the North. This is illustrated in Table 1-12, which shows estimated numbers and percentage migration of the cohort aged 65 and over at mid-decade, by state, between 1960 and 1970 and between 1970 and 1980. In each decade Florida experienced major in-migration—over 25 percent—followed by Arizona with over 20 percent. Nevada and New Mexico also experienced relatively high rates of immigration by the elderly. New York had the highest net migration to other states—238,000—followed by Illinois with 95,000, Pennsylvania with 85,000, and Ohio with 65,000.

Those who migrate will tend to be the more active and affluent and initially will make a positive contribution to the states to which they

Table 1-8. Projected growth of the total female population and the female
population aged 55 and over, 1990 to 2050*

Year	Female population (all ages)	Age groups			
		55-64	65-74	75-84	85 & over
		Numbers in thousands			
1990	128,139	11,180	10,172	6,494	2,393
2000	137,464	12,495	9,905	7,678	3,576
2010	145,209	18,128	11,206	7,621	4,761
2020	152,140	20,745	16,280	8,792	5,139
2030	156,902	17,450	18,644	12,861	6,140
2040	159,442	17,757	15,739	14,780	9,030
2050	160,070	19,068	16,110	12,577	11,247
		Percentage increase			
1990	-	-	-	-	-
2000	7.3	11.8	2.7	18.2	49.4
2010	5.6	45.1	13.1	-0.8	33.1
2020	4.8	14.4	45.3	15.4	7.9
2030	3.1	-16.0	4.0	46.3	19.5
2040	1.6	1.8	-15.6	15.0	47.0
2050	0.4	7.4	2.4	-15.0	25.0

* Middle-series projections.

Source: U.S. Bureau of the Census, Current Population Reports, Series P.25, No. 952,
Projections of the population of the United States by age, race and sex: 1983 to 2080.
Washington, D.C., U.S. Government Printing Office, 1984

retire. On the other hand, if they outlive their resources, they may present major future problems in need for assistance, both financial and personal. Other elderly individuals change residence within states, to more rural areas or smaller towns, while the poor and disabled tend to remain in their place of residence, often forming what have been described as "gerontic enclaves" in inner cities or other areas.[1]

Table 1-13 shows, by state, the population aged 65 and over and 85 and over, and the percentage of the total elderly population who are 85 and over. The national mean of the latter is 9.5 percent, with a range from less than 7 percent in Alaska to 12 percent in three predominantly rural states—Iowa, Nebraska, and South Dakota. This proportion will undoubtedly increase during the next two decades if current projections of national trends prove accurate.

Summary

Major changes have occurred in the size and age structure of the population during this century, with disproportionate growth in the elderly

Table 1-9. Projected growth of the total male population and the male population aged 55 and over, 1990 to 2050*

Year	Male population (all ages)	Age groups			
		55-64	65-74	75-84	85 & over
		Numbers in thousands			
1990	121,518	9,871	7,863	3,856	919
2000	130,491	11,272	7,773	4,640	1,350
2010	138,029	16,720	9,112	4,706	1,791
2020	144,457	19,554	13,574	5,695	1,942
2030	147,905	16,575	15,890	8,573	2,471
2040	149,118	16,960	13,533	10,093	3,804
2050	149,419	18,260	14,005	8,686	4,786
		Percentage increase			
1990	-	-	-	-	-
2000	7.4	14.2	-1.0	20.3	47.0
2010	6.2	48.3	17.2	1.4	32.7
2020	4.7	17.0	49.0	21.0	8.4
2030	2.4	-15.0	17.1	50.5	27.2
2040	0.8	2.3	-15.0	17.0	54.0
2050	0.2	7.7	3.5	-14.0	12.7

* Middle-series projections.

Source: U.S.Bureau of the Census, Current Population Reports, Series P-25, No. 952, Projections of the population of the United States by age, race and sex: 1983 to 2080. Washington, D.C., U.S. Government Printing Office, 1984.

population. In recent years the sector showing the highest rate of growth has been the very elderly, comprised of those aged 85 and over, and this growth is projected to continue.

Factors accounting for recent changes in population structure have been declining mortality rates and consequent increases in life expectancy for all age groups, including the very elderly; variations in the birthrate, from very high rates in the twenty years following World War II to less than two lifetime births per woman in recent years; and limited impact of net immigration on total population size and age structure compared with the early part of this century.

The aging of the "baby boom" generation, who will begin to reach age 65 in 2010, combined with predictions of a continuing decline in mortality rates and constant relatively low fertility levels, lead to projections of a major increase in the proportion of elderly individuals in the population well into the next century. There will be major percentage changes in the number of individuals in each elderly age group in successive decades after 2010 with the aging of the cohorts born between 1945 and 1965.

Table 1-10. Projections of the population aged 85 and over, 1990 to 2050*

Year	Population aged 85 & over	Age groups			
		85-89	90-94	95-99	100 & over
		Numbers in thousands			
1990	3,313	2,157	849	253	54
2000	4,926	3,025	1,355	438	108
2010	6,551	3,756	1,855	719	221
2020	7,081	3,587	2,158	975	361
2030	8,603	4,798	2,319	1,003	492
2040	12,834	7,012	3,777	1,448	597
2050	16,034	7,829	4,915	2,261	1,029
		Percentages			
1990	100.0	65.0	25.6	7.6	1.6
2000	100.0	61.4	27.5	8.9	2.2
2010	100.0	57.3	28.3	11.0	3.4
2020	100.0	51.0	30.5	13.8	5.1
2030	100.0	55.8	27.0	11.7	5.7
2040	100.0	55.0	29.4	11.3	4.7
2050	100.0	48.8	30.7	14.1	6.4

* Middle-series projections.

Source: U.S. Bureau of the Census, Current Population Reports, Series P-25, No. 952, Projections of the population of the United States, by age, race and sex: 1983 to 2080. Washington, D.C., U.S. Government Printing Office, 1984.

The geographical distribution of the elderly, both within and between states, could become of increasing importance with the aging of the population. There is wide variation, by state, in the distribution of the older population, brought about partly by patterns of migration on retirement. Some states in the North and Midwest are experiencing a net annual loss of elderly persons, leaving behind a disproportionate number of the poor and disabled and the very elderly. States such as Florida and Arizona have high annual rates of increase in the number and percentage of retired persons, with a high proportion of "younger elderly." Over time, however, the "Sunbelt states" will have a disproportionate number of very aged individuals, many with declining resources and an increasing need for long-term care.

Although there is every indication that the number of elderly persons will continue to grow, a small but persistent increase in the birthrate would lead to a rapid change in the age distribution of the population and a decline in the proportion of elderly. A reversal of present mortality trends would lead to a smaller than predicted increase in life expectancy and in the number of individuals of advanced old age.

Table 1-11. Total population and rank by state, population aged 65 and over and rank by state, elderly as a percentage of total population, 1980, and percentage increase in the elderly 1970-1980.

Numbers in thousands

State	Total population Number	Rank	Population aged 65 & over Number	Rank	Percent of total	Percentage increase 1970-80
United States	226,505	-	25,544	-	11.3	27.9
Alabama	3,890	22	440	24	11.3	35.8
Alaska	400	51	12	51	2.9	71.4
Arizona	2,178	29	307	25	11.3	90.7
Arkansas	2,286	33	312	2	13.7	31.6
California	23,669	1	2,415	34	10.2	34.8
Colorado	2,889	28	247	46	8.6	32.1
Connecticut	3,108	25	365	18	11.7	26.7
Delaware	595	48	59	36	10	34.1
District of Columbia	638	47	74	20	11.6	5.7
Florida	9,740	7	1,685	1	17.3	71.1
Georgia	5,464	13	517	41	9.5	41.6
Hawaii	965	39	76	49	7.9	72.7
Idaho	944	41	94	37	9.9	40.3
Illinois	11,418	5	1,261	29	11	15.8
Indiana	5,490	12	585	31	10.7	18.9
Iowa	2,913	27	387	4	13.3	10.9
Kansas	2,363	32	306	8	13	15.5
Kentucky	3,661	23	410	27	11.2	22
Louisiana	4,204	19	404	39	9.6	32.5
Maine	1,125	38	141	11	12.5	23.7
Maryland	4,216	18	396	42	9.4	32.9
Massachusetts	5,737	11	727	10	12.7	14.8
Michigan	9,258	8	912	38	9.8	21.8
Minnesota	4,077	21	480	17	11.8	17.9
Mississippi	2,521	31	289	21	11.5	30.8
Missouri	4,917	15	648	5	13.2	16.1
Montana	787	44	85	32	10.7	25
Nebraska	1,570	35	206	7	13.1	12.6
Nevada	799	43	66	47	8.2	113
New Hampshire	921	42	103	28	11.2	32.1
New Jersey	7,364	9	860	19	11.7	23.9
New Mexico	1,300	37	116	45	8.9	65.7
New York	17,557	2	2,161	13	12.3	10.8
North Carolina	5,874	10	602	35	10.2	46.1
North Dakota	653	46	80	14	12.3	21.1
Ohio	10,797	6	1,169	30	10.8	17.7
Oklahoma	3,025	26	376	12	12.4	25.8
Oregon	2,633	30	303	22	11.5	34.1
Pennsylvania	11,867	4	1,531	9	12.9	20.8
Rhode Island	947	40	127	3	13.4	22.1
South Carolina	3,119	24	287	44	9.2	51.1
South Dakota	690	45	91	6	13.2	13.8
Tennessee	4,591	17	518	26	11.3	35.6
Texas	14,228	3	1,371	40	9.6	38.8
Utah	1,461	36	109	50	7.5	41.4
Vermont	511	49	58	23	11.4	23.4
Virginia	5,346	14	505	43	9.4	38.7
Washington	4,130	20	431	33	10.4	31.7
West Virginia	1,950	34	238	15	12.2	22.7
Wisconsin	4,705	16	564	16	12	19.7
Wyoming	471	50	38	48	8	66.7

Source: Developments in Aging: Volume 1, 1982. A report of the Special Committee on Aging, United States Senate. Washington, D.C., U.S. Government Printing Office, 1983.

15

Table 1-12. Estimated net migration of the population cohort aged 65 and over at mid-decade, by state, 1970-1980 and 1960-1970.

State	1970 - 1980		1960 - 1970	
	Number	Rate**	Number	Rate**
United States	-113,000	-0.5	26,000	0.1
Alabama	2,000	0.6	3,000	1.2
Alaska	-2,000	-22.3	-2,000	-30.6
Arizona	50,000	23.6	24,000	21.2
Arkansas	11,000	4.0	9,000	4.2
California	57,000	2.7	92,000	5.9
Colorado	8,000	3.6	6,000	3.7
Connecticut	-5,000	-1.5	-	-
Delaware	-	0.7	-	1.0
District of Columbia	-13,000	-16.9	-12,000	0.6
Florida	317,000	25.9	205,000	29.3
Georgia	5,000	1.1	2,000	0.6
Hawaii	-3,000	-5.2	-6,000	-17.3
Idaho	3,000	4.0	1,000	1.7
Illinois	-95,000	-7.9	-62,000	-5.9
Indiana	-21,000	-3.9	-13,000	-2.7
Iowa	-1,000	-0.3	-	-
Kansas	2,000	0.6	4,000	1.7
Kentucky	-8,000	-2.0	-1,000	-0.4
Louisiana	-6,000	-1.8	-3,000	-1.0
Maine	3,000	2.3	-3,000	-2.7
Maryland	-12,000	-3.4	4,000	1.4
Massachusetts	-24,000	-3.5	-14,000	-2.3
Michigan	-50,000	-5.9	-29,000	-4.2
Minnesota	7,000	1.5	5,000	1.4
Mississippi	2,000	0.8	-4,000	-1.8
Missouri	-13,000	-2.2	-4,000	-0.7
Montana	-1,000	-1.6	-1,000	-1.5
Nebraska	2,000	1.1	4,000	2.2
Nevada	7,000	16.7	2,000	9.0
New Hampshire	4,000	4.9	1,000	0.9
New Jersey	-44,000	-5.6	-9,000	-1.4
New Mexico	8,000	9.6	2,000	2.5
New York	-238,000	-11.2	-137,000	-7.3
North Carolina	12,000	2.5	6,000	1.6
North Dakota	-	-0.1	-	-0.4
Ohio	-65,000	-5.9	-35,000	-3.7
Oklahoma	5,000	1.4	8,000	2.8
Oregon	11,000	4.1	10,000	4.8
Pennsylvania	85,000	6.1	63,000	5.1
Rhode Island	-2,000	-1.7	-2,000	-1.7
South Carolina	5,000	2.3	3,000	2.0
South Dakota	-	0.5	-	0.5
Tennessee	7,000	1.7	5,000	1.4
Texas	42,000	3.6	37,000	4.3
Utah	4,000	4.6	2,000	3.3
Vermont	1,000	2.0	-	-1.0
Virginia	2,000	0.5	2,000	0.6
Washington	11,000	2.9	3,000	1.2
West Virginia	10,000	4.5	8,000	4.4
Wisconsin	4,000	0.8	3,000	0.6
Wyoming	-2,000	-4.9	-1,000	-3.5

** Rate for 1970-80 represents net migration between 1970 and 1980 of the cohort 65 and over in 1975 as a percent of the population aged 65 and over in 1975. The same procedure for 1960-70.

Source: U.S. Bureau of the Census, Current Population Reports, Series P-23, No. 138, Demographic and socioeconomic aspects of aging in the United States. Washington, D.C., U.S. Government Printing Office, 1984

Table 1-13. Population aged 65 and over and 85 and over, and percentage of the total elderly population aged 85 and over, by state, 1981*

State	Population aged 65 & over	Population aged 85 & over	Percent of all elderly aged 85 & over
United States	25,492,531	2,440,571	9.5
Alabama	436,338	37,963	8.7
Alaska	11,798	780	6.6
Arizona	308,222	21,846	7.1
Arkansas	306,952	28,019	9.1
California	2,400,017	234,995	9.8
Colorado	250,151	26,074	10.4
Connecticut	370,905	38,811	10.5
Delaware	60,739	5,680	9.4
District of Columbia	70,074	8,055	11.5
Florida	1,626,466	128,205	7.9
Georgia	511,582	42,865	8.4
Hawaii	77,613	6,071	7.8
Idaho	97,707	8,957	9.2
Illinois	1,256,995	124,195	9.9
Indiana	590,198	56,868	9.6
Iowa	391,503	47,288	12.1
Kansas	307,320	35,377	11.5
Kentucky	407,365	37,548	9.2
Louisiana	385,639	37,380	9.7
Maine	144,618	15,416	10.7
Maryland	390,757	35,826	9.2
Massachusetts	723,376	81,324	11.2
Michigan	935,958	88,287	9.4
Minnesota	487,635	57,077	11.7
Mississippi	283,613	27,459	9.7
Missouri	644,610	65,941	10.2
Montana	87,670	9,301	10.6
Nebraska	207,141	25,083	12.1
Nevada	69,547	4,246	6.1
New Hampshire	105,766	10,490	9.9
New Jersey	866,691	79,645	9.2
New Mexico	118,353	10,115	8.5
New York	2,137,685	221,811	10.4
North Carolina	606,456	49,280	8.1
North Dakota	82,844	8,807	10.6
Ohio	1,182,861	115,930	9.8
Oklahoma	366,271	35,671	9.7
Oregon	308,877	30,425	9.9
Pennsylvania	1,543,787	141,335	9.1
Rhode Island	126,589	12,908	10.2
South Carolina	287,630	22,251	7.7
South Dakota	92,788	11,168	12.0
Tennessee	511,766	44,460	8.7
Texas	1,345,669	118,969	8.8
Utah	112,166	9,691	8.6
Vermont	59,314	6,389	10.8
Virginia	502,867	45,489	9.0
Washington	438,947	44,337	10.1
West Virginia	235,914	20,799	8.8
Wisconsin	578,070	59,906	10.4
Wyoming	38,711	3,758	9.7

* Estimates from Social Security data for 1981 differ slightly from U.S. Bureau of the Census data for 1980 used in Table 1-11 column 3.

Source: Social Security Administration, 1981 (unpublished data).

REFERENCES

1. U.S. Bureau of the Census, Current Population Reports, Series P-23, No. 138, Demographic and socioeconomic aspects of aging in the United States. Washington, D.C. U.S. Government Printing Office, 1984.
2. U.S. Bureau of the Census, 1980 Census of the Population, PC80-1-B1, General population characteristics: summary for the United States. Washington, D.C. U.S. Government Printing Office, May 1983.
3. U.S. Bureau of the Census, Current Population Reports, Series P-25, No. 952, Projections of the population of the United States by age, race and sex: 1983 to 2080, Washington, D.C. U.S. Government Printing Office, 1984.
4. National Center for Health Statistics: Health, United States, 1984. DHHS Pub. No. (PHS)85-1232, Public Health Service, Washington, D.C. U.S. Government Printing Office, December, 1984.
5. Siegel J. S., Passel J. S. New estimates of the number of centenarians in the United States. Journal of the American Statistical Association 71: 559–566, 1976.

2

Family Structure
and Living Arrangements

Despite widely held beliefs that most old people are geographically and socially isolated from their children and other relatives, and that "human service bureaucracies" are now chiefly responsible for the delivery of care to the elderly, studies over the past twenty years have shown that the family is still "the primary basis of security for adults in later life."[1-3] Even though different generations now tend to form separate households, most elderly people have frequent contact with children, grandchildren, siblings, and other relatives by blood or marriage. Furthermore, it has been demonstrated repeatedly that at any age or level of disability at least two people are being cared for in the community for every one who resides in a nursing home, with care being delivered predominantly by the family.[1,2,4,5]

Ill health often leads older people to live with their adult children if they can no longer maintain their own homes.[1] The low rate of institutionalization of elderly men has been attributed to their high rate of marriage and remarriage compared with elderly women and to the willingness and ability of wives to take care of their frequently older spouses, even when they are severely disabled.[6]

As might therefore be predicted, those without close family are statistically overrepresented in the nursing home population. Elderly widows and widowers are five times more likely to be institutionalized than married persons; those who have never married or are divorced or separated are ten times more likely to be institutionalized in old age. Fifty percent of nursing home residents have no children, and 20 percent have no immediate family.[5]

On the other hand, "the family" is not a static concept, and both its structure and function have changed over time. For instance, improved economic status of the elderly has facilitated independent living for each generation during the past thirty years, and continuing demographic, social, and economic changes are likely to generate further modification of family structure and behavior.

Life expectancy has increased constantly throughout the 20th century, and the first six decades showed a pattern of rising marriage rates accompanied by a decline in the proportion of childless women and in the mean maternal age at first birth. Recently, this has been replaced by one of lower marriage rates, a higher proportion of childless women, and a rise in the mean age at first birth.[7] In 1983 the proportion of women aged 30 to 34 who had never married was twice as high as in 1970.[8]

Marital and reproductive behavior is not predictable over time, but the average number of generations per family is expected to show a continuing increase because of declining mortality rates for all elderly age groups, so that in most families there will be two generations of elderly people—one aged 60 and over and one aged 80 and over. At the same time, it is projected that if fertility rates continue at present levels, the elderly in the 21st century will have fewer lineal descendents as well as siblings and other relatives.[7] These factors, together with the high divorce rates extant during the recent past, the increasing number of "one-parent families," and the rising proportion of women working outside the home, may well affect intergenerational relationships and lead to a decline of the family support system.

DATA SOURCES

Sources of information for the tables presented in this section are as follows.

The U.S. Bureau of the Census collects data on marital status and living arrangements through the decennial census of the population and also from population surveys published as Current Population Reports.[7-9] The other main information source is the National Center for Health Statistics, which collects state registration data on marriage and divorce through the National Vital Statistics System and additional data on family structure and living arrangements from national household and other surveys.[10-12]

Dependency Ratios

Potential family support for the elderly may be analyzed in terms of the size of the elderly population and the relative number of children, grandchildren, and other kin. Familial dependency ratios for the aged relate the population in a specified older age group at a given date to the population in a specified younger age group at the same date—corresponding approximately to the children of the former.[7]

It is estimated on the basis of 1970 census data that at the present time 78 percent of women aged 65 and over have at least one living child (80 percent of white women and 70 percent of black women). It is predicted that a larger proportion of the elderly will have a living child in 2000, but this trend will be reversed by 2025.[7]

Table 2-1 shows actual ratios between generations from 1930 to 1981 and projections to the year 2030. The upper half of the table relates the proportion of the population aged 65 to 79 to those aged 45 to 49; the lower half relates the population aged 80 and over to those aged 60 to 64 and the population aged 85 and over to those aged 65 to 69.

In 1981 there were 189 persons aged 65 to 79 for every 100 persons aged 45 to 49, compared with only 82 in 1930. It is projected that from 1985 onward this ratio will begin to decline steeply as the large birth cohorts of the postwar period begin to reach age 45, arriving at a low of 114 in 2005. The combination of the baby boom cohorts entering old age and the recent decline in fertility rates will mean a major rise in the ratio after 2010, reaching a peak of 252 in 2025.

Increasing life expectancy means that many persons in extreme old age depend on children who are themselves elderly. The ratio between these elderly cohorts is important in terms of the ability of one generation to provide support for the next.

As shown in the lower half of Table 2-1, there were 21 persons aged 80 and over for every 100 persons 60 to 64 years in 1930 but, by 1981, the ratio was two and a half times greater, at 53. It is projected that by 2000 there will be 96 individuals aged 80 and over for every 100 aged 60 to 64. Thereafter the ratio is expected to decline, but it should peak again to approximately 1:1 in 2030. The ratio of individuals aged 85 and over to those aged 65 to 69 increased from 10 in 1930 to 27 in 1981 and is projected to reach a peak of 61 in 2005.

Marital Status

The proportion of married men and married women is highest and approximately equal at about age 35. After age 45, the proportion of married men tends to be much higher than the proportion of married women because of the lower rate of widowhood of men and their higher rate of remarriage following divorce.

Tables 2-2 and 2-3 show the distribution of the male and female populations aged 55 and over by marital status and age, from 1960 to 1981, with projections to 1995. In all older age groups more men than women are married and, while the proportion married declines and the proportion widowed increases with advancing age for both sexes, there is a dramatic difference between the marital experience of men and women. In 1981 the proportion of men who were married with spouse present was 82 percent for those aged 55 to 64, 80 percent for those 65 to 74, and 70 percent for those aged 75 and over. By comparison, the proportions were only 67 percent, 48 percent, and 22 percent for women in the same age groups.

Table 2-1. Familial aged dependency ratios, with one elderly generation and with two elderly generations, actual and projected series, 1930-2030.

With one elderly generation

Year	Ratio*
Estimates	Actual series
1930	82
1940	95
1950	166
1960	129
1970	135
1980	185
1981	189
	Projections**
1985	192
1990	174
1995	142
2000	126
2005	114
2010	126
2015	171
2020	220
2025	252
2030	241

*Ratios are: Population 65 to 79 years/Population 45 to 49 years x 100

With Two Elderly Generations

Year	Ratio A (a)	Ratio B (b)
Estimates	Actual series	Actual series
1930 (c)	21	10
1940 (c)	24	10
1950 (c)	29	12
1960 (c)	36	15
1970	43	20
1980	52	26
1981	53	27
	Projections**	Projections**
1985	57	30
1990	71	35
2000	96	56
2005	91	61
2010	77	58
2015	69	49
2020	65	44
2025	74	43
2030	101	49

(a) Population 80 and over/Population 60 to 64 years x 100

(b) Population 85 and over/Population 65 to 69 years x 100

(c) Based on census data and relates to April 1.

** Middle-series projections.

(Figures are shown for July 1 of the year indicated. Familial aged dependency ratios relate a group of elderly or aged persons to a group of younger adults of appropriate ages in a parent-child relationship.)

Source: U.S. Bureau of the Census, Current Population Reports, Series P-23, No. 138, Demographic & socioeconomic aspects of aging in the United States. Washington, D.C., U.S. Government Printing Office, 1984.

Table 2-2. Distribution of the male population aged 55 years and over, by marital status and by age, 1960 to 1981 with projections to 1995.

Marital status and year	Age groups		
	55-64	65-74	75 & over
1960			
Total	100.0	100.0	100.0
Single	7.9	6.7	7.8
Married	82.4	78.9	59.1
Spouse present	79.0	76.2	56.5
Spouse absent	3.4	2.7	2.6
Widowed	6.2	12.7	31.6
Divorced	3.5	1.7	1.5
1970			
Total	100.0	100.0	100.0
Single	7.8	8.0	6.6
Married	85.2	78.0	64.3
Spouse present	82.3	75.2	60.4
Spouse absent	2.9	2.8	3.9
Widowed	4.1	11.3	27.7
Divorced	3.0	2.7	1.4
1975			
Total	100.0	100.0	100.0
Single	6.5	4.3	5.5
Married	85.0	83.8	70.0
Spouse present	81.8	81.8	68.2
Spouse absent	3.2	2.0	1.8
Widowed	4.0	8.8	23.3
Divorced	4.5	3.1	1.2
1981			
Total	100.0	100.0	100.0
Single	5.1	4.9	3.5
Married	84.7	83.0	72.0
Spouse present	81.7	80.6	69.7
Spouse absent	3.1	2.4	2.2
Widowed	4.0	8.2	22.1
Divorced	6.1	3.9	2.5
1990 *			
Total	100.0	100.0	100.0
Single	4.8	5.6	5.0
Married, spouse present	81.5	77.8	68.6
Other ever married**	13.7	16.5	26.4
1995 *			
Total	100.0	100.0	100.0
Single	4.4	5.3	4.7
Married, spouse present	81.1	78.4	70.9
Other ever married**	14.5	16.3	24.5

* Middle-range projections, March 1978.

** Comprises divorced, widowed, and married, spouse absent.

Source: U.S. Bureau of the Census, Current Population Reports, Series P-23, No. 138, Demographic and socioeconomic aspects of aging in the United States. Washington, D.C., U.S. Government Printing Office, 1984.

Table 2-3. Distribution of the female population aged 55 years and over, by marital status and by age, 1960 to 1981 with projections to 1995.

Marital status and year	Age groups		
	55–64	65–74	75 & over
1960			
Total	100.0	100.0	100.0
Single	6.5	8.4	8.6
Married	65.8	45.6	21.8
Spouse present	62.9	43.5	20.6
Spouse absent	2.9	2.1	1.2
Widowed	24.5	44.4	68.3
Divorced	3.2	1.7	1.2
1970			
Total	100.0	100.0	100.0
Single	6.8	7.8	7.5
Married	67.4	45.2	21.0
Spouse present	63.8	43.5	19.1
Spouse absent	3.6	1.6	1.9
Widowed	21.2	44.0	70.3
Divorced	4.6	3.0	1.3
1975			
Total	100.0	100.0	100.0
Single	5.1	5.8	5.8
Married	69.3	49.1	23.4
Spouse present	66.7	47.3	22.3
Spouse absent	2.6	1.8	1.1
Widowed	20.3	41.9	69.4
Divorced	5.3	3.3	1.5
1981			
Total	100.0	100.0	100.0
Single	4.2	5.4	6.2
Married	70.3	50.1	23.3
Spouse present	67.1	48.3	21.8
Spouse absent	3.2	1.8	1.5
Widowed	18.4	40.1	68.2
Divorced	7.1	4.4	2.3
1990 *			
Total	100.0	100.0	100.0
Single	3.6	5.7	5.7
Married, spouse present	70.3	47.7	20.0
Other ever married**	26.1	46.5	74.3
1995 *			
Total	100.0	100.0	100.0
Single	3.1	5.3	5.4
Married, spouse present	71.8	48.8	20.5
Other ever married**	25.1	45.9	74.2

* Middle-range projections, March 1978.

** Comprises divorced, widowed, and married, spouse absent.

Source: U.S. Bureau of the Census, Current Population Reports, Series P-23, No. 138, Demographic and socioeconomic aspects of aging in the United States. Washington, D.C., U.S. Government Printing Office, 1984.

Between 1960 and 1981 the proportion of men aged 75 and over who were married increased from 59 to 72 percent and the proportion widowed declined from 32 to 22 percent. By contrast, during the same period the percentage of women aged 75 and over who were married ranged from 21 to 23 percent and the proportion widowed also remained constant at 68 to 70 percent.

As shown in Tables 2-4 and 2-5, there are marked differences in marital status between the black and white elderly populations, with blacks being less likely than whites to be married with spouse present in all old age groups. Forty-two percent of black men aged 75 and over in 1983 were widowed, single, or divorced compared with 27 percent of white men, and 80 percent of black women were in the same situation compared with 75 percent of white women.[8]

The continuing differences in life expectancy between men and women and the tendency of men to marry women younger than themselves and to remarry when widowed or divorced seem likely to ensure that the present pattern will persist. Marital status is an important indicator of the

Table 2-4. Marital status of the total white population and the white population aged 55 and over, 1981.

Numbers in thousands

| | | Age groups | | |
	Total population*	55-64	65-74	75 & over
Total	154,108	19,622	14,376	8,858
Single	37,929	802	787	455
Widowed	11,035	2,020	3,619	4,369
Married, spouse absent	3,709	363	197	96
Married, spouse present	91,686	15,289	9,133	3,718
Divorced	9,749	1,148	640	220

Percentage

Total	100.0	100.0	100.0	100.0
Single	25.0	4.0	5.5	5.1
Widowed	7.2	10.3	25.2	49.3
Married, spouse absent	2.4	2.0	1.2	1.1
Married, spouse present	59.5	78.0	64.0	42.0
Divorced	6.3	6.0	4.5	2.5

*Total white population aged 15 years and over.

Source: U.S. Bureau of the Census, Current Population Reports, Series P-20, No. 372, Marital status and living arrangements: March 1981. Washington, D.C., U.S. Government Printing Office, 1982.

Table 2-5. Marital status of the total black population and the black population aged
55 and over, 1981.

Numbers in thousands

	Total population*	Age groups 55-64	65-74	75 & over
Total	19,944	1,960	1,343	780
Single	7,558	125	46	18
Widowed	1,593	335	494	466
Married, spouse absent	1,603	227	91	26
Married, spouse present	7,066	1,063	640	240
Divorced	1,624	211	73	30

Percentage

Total	100.0	100.0	100.0	100.0
Single	39.0	6.4	3.4	2.3
Widowed	8.2	17.1	37.0	60.0
Married, spouse absent	8.2	12.0	7.0	3.3
Married, spouse present	36.3	54.0	48.0	31.0
Divorced	8.4	11.0	5.4	3.8

*Total black population aged 15 years and over.

Source: U.S. Bureau of the Census, Current Population Reports, Series P-20, No.
372, Marital status and living arrangements: March 1981. Washington, D.C., U.S.
Government Printing Office, 1982.

need for institutional care in later life. Fifty-four percent of the elderly
noninstitutionalized population is married;[9] in 1977 only 12 percent of
the elderly nursing home population was married.[10]

Divorce Rates

A factor liable to have a major and continuing impact on family structure
and relationships is the high rate of divorce. The annual total of divorces
tripled between 1961 and 1981, from 414,000 to 1,213,000, and the estimated number of children involved in divorce has been more than 1 million every year since 1972.[11]

The overall divorce ratio rose from 47 divorced persons per 1,000 currently married persons with spouse present to 114 between 1970 and
1983 (see Table 2-6). Divorce ratios are lower for men than for women—
91 compared with 137—because of the higher rate of remarriage of
divorced men; the ratios are higher among blacks than whites, with black
women having the highest ratio of all (297 per 1,000). Divorce ratios
decline with age, but the greatest difference between male and female

Table 2-6. Divorced persons per 1,000 married persons with spouse present by age, sex and race, 1960, 1970, 1980 and 1983.

Year & sex	Age groups				
	Under 30	30-34	35-44	45-64	65 & over
Both sexes					
1983	111	141	147	103	70
1980	96	131	122	91	64
1970	38	45	48	53	47
1960	23	30	35	46	32
Male					
1983	98	126	118	81	43
1980	78	108	101	70	48
1970	28	33	32	40	32
1960	16	23	26	39	24
Female					
1983	121	155	177	126	106
1980	108	153	143	112	89
1970	46	56	64	66	69
1960	28	37	44	53	44

Year & sex	Race			
	All races	White	Black	Spanish origin
Both sexes				
1983	114	106	230	114
1980	100	92	203	98
1970	47	44	83	61
1960	35	33	62	NA
Male				
1983	91	87	164	78
1980	79	74	149	64
1970	35	32	62	40
1960	28	27	45	NA
Female				
1983	137	126	297	149
1980	120	110	258	132
1970	60	56	104	81
1960	42	38	78	NA

Source: U.S. Bureau of the Census, Current Population Reports Series P-20, No. 389, Marital status and living arrangements, March, 1983.   Washington, D.C., U.S. Government Printing Office, 1984.

ratios is for those aged 65 and over—43 for men compared with 106 for women.

There was a 3.5-percent drop in the total number of divorces and a 6-percent decrease in the number of children involved in divorce in 1982 compared with 1981, but the divorce rate was still nearly 22 per 1,000 married women compared with less than 10 in 1962.[11]

Living Arrangements

There was a 75-percent increase in the number of persons living alone between 1970 and 1981 and, while this was largely attributable to single and divorced persons and to those in the age group 35 to 44, there was a 30-percent increase in the number of men aged 65 and over living alone and a 55-percent increase for women in this age group.[9]

In 1975 it was estimated that four out of five noninstitutionalized persons aged 65 and over had living children but, while this proportion had remained stable for 20 years, the number who lived in the same households had declined from 36 percent in 1957 to 18 percent in 1975.[1]

Table 2-7 shows the living arrangements of the elderly in 1970 and 1983. Since 1970 there has been more change in the living arrangements of the noninstitutionalized population aged 75 and over than for those aged 65 to 74. For the older elderly, the proportion living with relatives (in families) declined from 64 percent in 1970 to 59 percent in 1983. Seven out of ten of 5.8 million persons aged 75 and over living in families in 1983 were husbands and wives maintaining their own households versus six out of ten in 1970. Forty percent maintained their own household alone or shared it with someone unrelated to them, compared with 34 percent in 1970.[8]

The population aged 65 to 74 showed no change between 1970 and 1983 in the proportion living with relatives (72 percent in 1983, 73 percent in 1970). Those living as husbands and wives grew only slightly, from 58 percent to 62 percent. The 26 percent who lived alone or with nonrelatives in 1983 showed no significant change from 23 percent in 1970.[8]

Changes over time in the living arrangements of the male and female populations aged 65 and over are shown in Table 2-8. Between 1965 and 1981, the percentage of men aged 65 to 74 living alone remained essentially the same, at 11 to 12 percent, and the percentage of men aged 75 and over living alone increased modestly, from 16 to 19 percent. In contrast, the percentage of women aged 65 to 74 living alone rose from 28 to 34 percent, and there was a 50-percent increase in the proportion of women aged 75 and over living alone—from 30 to 45 percent. Other survey data from 1979 and 1980 showed that the proportion of men and women living with relatives other than a spouse increased from 9 percent of men and 24 percent of women in the age range 75 to 84 to 22 percent

Table 2-7. Living arrangements of the elderly, 1970 and 1983

Numbers in thousands

	1983			1970		
	Total	Age group		Total	Age group	
		65-74	75 & over		65-74	75 & over
Total persons:	25,737	15,981	9,756	19,061	12,093	6,968
In Families						
Married, spouse present.	7,937	5,467	2,470	5,749	4,011	1,738
Other	1,658	917	741	1,456	787	669
Spouse of householder	5,855	4,373	1,482	3,843	2,986	857
Other relative	1,872	814	1,057	2,294	1,079	1,215
Not in families*						
Householder	8,074	4,219	3,855	5,295	2,947	2,348
Living alone	7,856	4,095	3,761	5,071	2,815	2,256
Nonrelative of householder	242	138	104	290	190	100
In group quarters	101	54	47	137	95	42
Percentage:	100.0	100.0	100.0	100.0	100.0	100.0
In families	67.3	72.4	58.9	70.0	73.3	64.3
Married, spouse present	30.8	34.2	25.3	30.2	33.2	24.9
Other	6.4	5.7	7.6	7.6	6.5	9.6
Spouse of householder	22.7	27.4	15.2	20.2	24.7	12.3
Other relative	7.3	5.1	10.8	12.0	8.9	17.4
Not in families *	32.7	27.6	41.1	30.0	26.7	35.7
Living alone	30.5	25.6	38.6	26.6	23.3	32.4
Nonrelative of householder	0.9	0.9	1.1	1.5	1.6	1.4
In group quarters	0.4	0.3	0.5	0.7	0.8	0.6

* Includes persons in unrelated subfamilies.

Source: U.S. Bureau of the Census, Current Population Reports, Series P-20, No. 389, Marital status and living arrangements: March 1983. Washington, D.C., U.S. Government Printing Office, 1984.

Table 2-8. Living arrangements of the male population aged 65 and over, and living arrangements of the female population aged 65 and over, 1965, 1975 and 1981.

Numbers in thousands

	Males		Females	
	Age groups			
1981	65 to 74	75 & over	65 to 74	75 & over
Number	6,874	3,632	8,981	6,555
In households	6,727	3,375	8,780	5,785
Living alone	761	689	3,075	2,959
With spouse	5,429	2,354	4,247	1,263
With other person	537	332	1,458	1,563
Not in households	147	257	201	770
Percentage	100.0	100.0	100.0	100.0
In households	97.9	92.9	97.8	88.3
Living alone	11.1	19.0	34.2	45.1
With spouse	79.0	64.8	47.3	19.3
With other person	7.8	9.1	16.2	23.8
Not in households	2.1	7.1	2.2	11.7
1975				
Percentage	100.0	100.0	100.0	100.0
In households	97.1	92.7	97.5	90.0
Living alone	12.1	18.2	32.9	40.6
With spouse	79.6	63.3	46.2	20.1
With other person	5.4	11.2	18.4	29.3
Not in households	2.9	7.3	2.5	10.0
1965				
Percentage	100.0	100.0	100.0	100.0
In households	97.5	93.6	97.4	92.0
Living alone	11.7	15.7	27.9	29.9
With spouse	75.3	54.0	43.3	19.0
With other person	10.5	23.9	26.1	43.1
Not in households	2.5	6.4	2.6	8.0

Source: U.S. Bureau of the Census, Current Population Reports, Series P-23, No. 138, Demographic and socioeconomic aspects of aging in the Aspects of Aging in the United States. Washington, D.C., U.S. Government Printing Office, 1984

of men and 44 percent of women aged 85 and over.[12] This is indicative of the importance of the family at the present time, in caring for the dependent elderly.

While the percentage of households maintained by married couples in which the householder is aged 65 and over is projected to change very

Table 2-9. Number and percentage of the total population aged 65 and over in long-term institutions, 1950, 1960, 1970 and 1980.

	1950	1960	1970	1980
		Number		
All institutions	378,515	607,917	959,837	1,336,502
Nursing homes	217,536	387,953	795,807	1,232,958
Mental institutions	145,530	182,602	123,770	51,105
T.B. & chronic disease hospitals	15,449	37,362	40,260	52,439
		Percentage		
All institutions	3.05	3.64	4.78	5.2
Nursing homes	1.77	2.32	3.96	4.8
Mental institutions	1.19	1.09	0.62	0.2
T.B. & chronic disease hospitals	0.13	0.22	0.2	0.2

Source: U.S. Bureau of the Census. Decennial Censuses of Population, 1950, 1960, 1970, 1980. (Personal communication).

little up to 1995, the proportion of households in which the householder is an elderly female living alone or with nonrelatives is expected to increase substantially, particularly for those aged 75 and over.[7]

Institutionalized Elderly

Information on the total institutionalized population is collected in the decennial censuses of the population. The population in long-term institutions includes persons under care or custody in places such as homes for the aged and hospitals for the physically or mentally handicapped or for chronic disease patients.

As shown in Table 2-9, based on census data since 1950, the proportion of elderly in long-term institutions has shown a slight progressive increase in each decade. There was a 19-percent increase in the percentage of the elderly in institutions between 1950 and 1960, a 31-percent increase between 1960 and 1970, but only an 8-percent increase from 1970 to 1980. In 1950, 3.05 percent of the elderly were in institutions; by 1980 this had increased to 5.2 percent.

In the 1980 census 92 percent of the 1.3 million persons aged 65 and over in institutions were in homes for the aged. The corresponding proportion in 1970 was 82 percent of 968,000 institutionalized elderly.

Data on the number and percent of individuals living in "life care communities" and other recent housing developments for the elderly are not available.

Summary

Although recent survey data show that most elderly people have frequent contact with their children, siblings, and other relatives and that the family is the major care provider for the dependent elderly, demographic, social, and economic trends all indicate that there may be less family support for the elderly in the future. As life expectancy increases, family size is diminishing, there is a high rate of disruption in family relationships, and generations are becoming more physically isolated from each other.

Increasing life expectancy for the elderly combined with lower fertility rates among younger age groups means that each family is tending to have more generations, but that in the future the elderly will have fewer lineal descendents and other relatives.

Although more women are now marrying than in the past, the greater longevity of women and the higher rates of remarriage for men, usually to younger women, following widowhood or divorce means that a high and increasing number of elderly women are without spouses.

During the past twenty years, there have been major increases in divorce rates, in the number of children involved in divorce, and in the ratio of divorced to married persons. Although divorce rates may now have reached a plateau, they are still higher than previously existed. The long-term effects of these disruptions in family relationships is not yet known, but it is difficult to predict that they will not weaken the traditional intergenerational support networks.

These factors, combined with the increasing labor force participation of women, who have traditionally provided care to elderly relatives, all indicate that as the proportion of elderly persons in the population increases, the amount of available family support will decline.

An additional factor is the increasing physical separation of generations within the same family, even without migration to other states, leading to an increasing proportion of individuals living alone with advancing age. Although the increase for men has been modest, the proportion of elderly women living alone is now 50 percent higher than in 1965 and is expected to increase substantially, particularly for the very elderly. The tendency for different generations to form separate households is indicative of increasing economic independence, but it also creates problems in the longer term as life expectancy increases and individuals either outlive their resources or become increasingly frail and dependent or both.

There has been a progressive increase in the proportion of elderly persons living in long-term institutions between 1950 and 1980, and there is likely to be an increasing demand for private or publicly financed care for the elderly, particularly women, either in the home, in nursing homes, or in other communities for the elderly.

REFERENCES

1. Shanas E. Social myth as hypothesis: the case of the family relations of old people. The Gerontologist 19: 6: 3–9, 1979.
2. Shanas E. The Family as a social support system in old age. The Gerontologist 19: 2: 169–174, 1979.
3. Treas J. Family support systems for the aged: some social and demographic considerations. The Gerontologist 17: 6: 486–491, 1977.
4. Department of Health and Human Services, Office of the Assistant Secretary for Planning and Evaluation, 1984. Working Papers on Long-Term Care. Prepared for the 1980 Under Secretary's Task Force on Long Term Care, Washington, D.C. U.S. Government Printing Office, 1984.
5. Doty P. Family care of the elderly: is it declining? Can public policy promote it? Office of Legislation and Policy. Health Care Financing Administration, (working paper), 1984.
6. Fengler A. P., Goodrich B. A. Wives of elderly, disabled men: the hidden patients. The Gerontologist 19: 2: 175–183, 1979.
7. U.S. Bureau of the Census, Current Population Reports, Series P-23, No. 138, Demographic and socioeconomic aspects of aging in the United States. Washington, D.C. U.S. Government Printing Office, 1984.
8. U.S. Bureau of the Census, Current Population Reports, Series P-20, No. 389, Marital status and living arrangements: March 1983. Washington, D.C. U.S. Government Printing Office, 1984.
9. U.S. Bureau of the Census, Current Population Reports, Series P-20, No. 372, Marital Status and Living Arrangements: March 1981. Washington, D.C. U.S. Government Printing Office, 1982.
10. National Center for Health Statistics, National Nursing Home Survey, 1977, Summary for the United States, Vital and Health Statistics, Series 13, No. 43. DHEW Pub. No. (PHS)79-1794. Public Health Service. U.S. Government Printing Office, July 1979.
11. National Center for Health Statistics: Advance report of final divorce statistics, 1982. Monthly Vital Statistics Report, Vol. 33, No. 11, Supp. DHHS Pub. No. (PHS)85-1120, Public Health Service, Hyattsville, Md., Feb. 28, 1985.
12. National Center for Health Statistics. Feller B. A. Need for care among the noninstitutionalized elderly. Health, United States, 1983. DHHS Pub. No. (PHS)84-1232. Public Health Service, Washington, D.C. U.S. Government Printing Office, December, 1983.

3

Income of the Elderly

There is a clear pattern of declining income with advancing age, although little hard data on total assets of the elderly are available. Income of the elderly may be derived from the following sources: Social Security benefits; private, government employee, or other pensions; income from assets; public assistance; or earnings from employment. Older persons who work full time tend to have incomes similar to younger persons of the same race and sex[1] and, for the total population aged 65 and over, earnings from employment provide a higher percentage of income than all other sources except Social Security.[2] The average income of individuals aged 85 and over is 36 percent less than for those aged 65 to 69, the decline being largely associated with a 74-percent decrease in labor force participation between the two age cohorts.[3]

Before the passage of the Social Security Act in 1935, the primary sources of financial support for all individuals, including the elderly, were employment income and the family. Federal programs that have been developed under the umbrella of the 1935 act to provide income or income support are of two types.

1. Social insurance entitlements under the Old Age Survivors and Disability Insurance (OASDI) and Medicare programs for those who qualify on the basis of age and contributions made by, or on behalf of, beneficiaries.
2. Means-tested public assistance benefits in cash or in kind, such as Supplemental Security Income, food stamps, and Medicaid.

Social Security Income

The Social Security system is designed to provide a foundation of insurance protection and retirement benefit accumulation throughout each individual's working career. It shares the basic cost of supporting the retired generation among those still working.[1]

Mandatory contributions for Old Age Insurance were first collected in 1937, with coverage confined to private sector workers in commerce and industry, accounting for a little over 40 percent of the work force. Coverage has been gradually extended over time to include 95 percent of all workers.[1]

The Federal Old Age and Survivors Insurance Trust Fund was established on January 1, 1940, as a separate account in the U.S. Treasury, and all financial operations of this program are handled through the fund. The Federal Disability Insurance Trust Fund is another separate account, established in 1956. The major sources of receipts for these two funds are from contributions paid by workers and their employers and by individuals with self-employment income in work covered by the OASDI program. Contributions are collected by the Internal Revenue Service and deposited in the general fund of the Treasury, from which estimated payments are then made to the OASDI funds and to the Medicare Hospital Insurance (HI) fund. The amount of benefits to which an individual, or his or her spouse and children, may become entitled is based on the individual's taxable lifetime earnings.[4]

The normal retirement age for full benefits is 65, but individuals may elect to receive reduced benefits at the age of 62. Increased payments or retirement credits are payable to individuals who delay retirement past the age of 65.

Amendments to the Social Security Act in 1972 increased all benefits by 20 percent and initiated the indexing of benefits. This was implemented in 1975; since then, the consumer price index (CPI) has been used to index Social Security payments, thus maintaining the purchasing power of this part of elderly income.[1]

The 1983 Social Security Amendments, Public Law 98-21, modified the existing provisions in the interests of ensuring the financial stability of the system into the next century. Significant changes included a gradual increase in the normal retirement age from 65 to 67 between 2000 and 2022 and a gradual increase in retirement credits after 1990 for those deferring the receipt of benefits beyond normal retirement age. In addition, in 1984 Social Security payments became subject to taxation for the first time for those with incomes above certain base amounts.

Supplemental Security Income

The Supplemental Security Income (SSI) program is a federally administered income assistance program authorized by Title XVI of the Social Security Act in 1972 and implemented in 1974. The SSI program replaced four other titles of the Social Security Act, transferring basic administrative responsibilities for public assistance from the states to the federal government and providing a national minimum income level for the aged, blind, and disabled poor who meet both asset and income tests.[5]

Federal payments are based on the difference between the individual's income and the minimum income level established nationally. Payment levels are set for individuals and for couples living independently and are adjusted for those in other living arrangements. As with Social Security benefits, since 1975 payments have been adjusted annually to increases in the cost of living.

The law requires a benefit reduction of one third for those who live in another person's household and who receive support and maintenance from that person or persons. If an individual enters an institution, where care is primarily financed by Medicaid, SSI payment is reduced to $25 per month. SSI payments may be made to persons in publicly operated community residences serving not more than 16 persons and to residents of public emergency shelters for up to three months per year.[5]

Eligibility for SSI is restricted to qualified persons who have assets of less than $1,500 for individuals living alone or $2,250 for married couples living alone. This has not changed since the beginning of the program in 1974. The value of a person's home is not counted as a resource for SSI eligiblity, but regulations establish limits on the value of automobiles, household goods and personal effects, life insurance policies, and other assets that can be excluded from consideration in determining eligibility.[1]

Mandatory minimum state supplementation of federal benefits are required, by law, to maintain the December 1973 income levels of former public assistance recipients who were transferred to the SSI program. Compliance with this provision is required for states to maintain their eligibility for Title XIX (Medicaid) federal matching funds. The SSI program also allows states to establish their own minimum income levels, above the federal standards, through supplemental payments that are not counted as income in calculating federal benefits. States with optional programs supplement recipients' federal payments to bring incomes up to the higher state minimum level. Recipients may have enough income to put them above the federal level but below the state level, in which case individuals would be eligible for state payments only. Optional state supplementary payments may vary across recipient categories (i.e., aged, blind, disabled) and may also vary by geographic area and living arrangement.[6]

In 1984, all but eight states (Arkansas, Georgia, Kansas, Mississippi, North Dakota, Tennessee, Texas, and West Virginia) had some form of optional supplementation. North Dakota and West Virginia did make payments for "special needs" of aged, blind, and disabled SSI recipients.[6] A number of states use SSI payments to provide nonmedical institutional care for eligible individuals (see Chapter 9).

States may administer their own supplement programs or arrange with the Social Security Administration for joint administration with the federal benefits.

Other Federal Assistance Programs

In addition to cash contributions, the government provides benefits to the elderly poor in the form of medical care, food stamps, publicly owned or subsidized rental housing, and energy assistance.

In all but 15 states, persons receiving federal or state SSI payments are automatically eligible for Medicaid. Where Medicaid eligibility standards are more restrictive, Medicaid applicants may deduct their medical expenses from their income for purposes of eligibility determination.[5]

Food stamp program benefits are federally established and vary according to household size and according to whether a household has special expenses for medical care or related needs. SSI beneficiaries may qualify for food stamps if they meet the income and asset requirements. California and Wisconsin have chosen to increase state SSI payments in lieu of food stamps.[5]

DATA SOURCES

Sources of information for the tables presented in this chapter are as follows.

Information on income of the elderly is obtained by the Bureau of the Census in the decennial census of the population.

Labor force participation ratios by age may be computed from estimates made by the Bureau of Labor Statistics of the U.S. Department of Labor.

The annual report of the Social Security Administration provides data on the Social Security population, with actual and projected dependency ratios and comparisons between the number of beneficiaries and the number of workers covered by the Old Age Survivors and Disability Insurance.[4]

Since 1941, the Social Security Administration has made periodic surveys of the economic situation of the aged as part of a statutory mandate to measure the effectiveness of the Social Security program.[7,8]

Income Sources and Distribution

In 1978 16 percent of the elderly lived exclusively on Social Security payments; another 26 percent received more than 90 percent of their income from these benefits.[9] As shown in Table 3-1, income from Social Security increases as a proportion of the total income of the elderly, from 2 percent for those aged 55 to 61 to 50 percent for those aged 80 and over. At the same time, income from earnings declines. Eighty percent of income is derived from earnings for those aged 55 to 61, compared with 4 percent for those aged 80 and over.

It is theorized that individuals save during their working life so that they can maintain consumption after retirement by "dissaving" or spending down their assets.[3] The percentage of income from assets for elderly age groups, shown in Table 3-1, tends to confirm this theory. Asset income increased progressively, from 9 percent for those aged 55 to 61 to 30 percent or more for those aged 73 to 79 and 80 and over in 1982.

Table 3-1. Percentage distribution of money income from particular sources for aged units* 55 and over, 1980 and 1982.

	Age group					
1980	55-61	62-64	65-67	68-72	73-79	80 & over
Percent of income from:	100.0	100.0	100.0	100.0	100.0	100.0
Social Security	2.0	12.0	28.0	38.0	44.0	50.0
Govt. employee pensions	4.0	6.0	8.0	7.0	6.0	7.0
Private pensions	2.0	5.0	7.0	8.0	6.0	5.0
Other pensions		1.0	1.0	1.0	1.0	1.0
Earnings	80.0	60.0	34.0	20.0	13.0	4.0
Income from assets	8.0	12.0	18.0	22.0	26.0	25.0
Public assistance	1.0	1.0	1.0	1.0	2.0	3.0
Other	3.0	2.0	3.0	1.0		3.0
1982						
Percent of income from:	100.0	100.0	100.0	100.0	100.0	100.0
Social Security	2.0	13.0	28.0	38.0	44.0	48.0
Govt. employee pensions	4.0	6.0	7.0	7.0	7.0	7.0
Private pensions	2.0	5.0	7.0	7.0	6.0	4.0
Other pensions	1.0	1.0	2.0	2.0	2.0	3.0
Earnings	79.0	58.0	35.0	19.0	10.0	4.0
Income from assets	9.0	14.0	18.0	24.0	30.0	31.0
Public assistance	1.0	1.0	1.0	1.0	1.0	2.0
Other	2.0	2.0	2.0	2.0	2.0	2.0

* An aged unit is a married couple living together or a nonmarried person.

Source: U.S. Department of Health and Human Services, Income of the population 55 and over, 1980. SSA Publication No. 13-11871, Social Security Administration, Office of Policy, Office of Research and Statistics. U.S. Government Printing Office, January 1983, and and U.S. Department of Health and Human Services, Income of the population 55 and over, 1982. SSA Publication No. 13-11871, Social Security Administration, Office of Policy, Office of Research and Statistics. U.S. Government Printing Office, March, 1984.

Income tends to increase with age until about age 55, when significant numbers of individuals begin to retire. As shown in Table 3-2, the median income for both married couples living together and for nonmarried persons declines progressively for each elderly age group compared with those aged 55 to 61. At age 80, the median income in 1980 was only 29 percent of the median income for those aged 55 to 61, although it had increased to 31 percent in 1982. Median income at all ages is highest for married couples and for men compared with nonmarried persons and women.

Tables 3-3 and 3-4 compare the income distribution for men and women and blacks and whites. Income becomes progressively more skewed toward the lower end of the distribution with advancing age for all sex and race categories. Those with the highest proportion of incomes below $6,000 per year in all elderly age groups are blacks and females but, by age 75, the majority of all individuals in 1979 had incomes of less than $6,000. Sixty-five percent of the white population, 87 percent of the black population, 53 percent of males of all races, and 76 percent of females of all races were in this income category.

Table 3-5 shows the median income for households with householders aged 65 and over by race and by state in 1979. The median income for households with an elderly white householder was 35 percent higher than for those with an elderly black householder, $12,671 compared with $9,356. Median income ranged from a high of $30,396 in the District of Columbia to a low of $9,409 in Arkansas for elderly white households. For elderly black households the range was from a high of $13,711 in the District of Columbia to a low of $6,091 in Arkansas.

Poverty Rates

In 1972 the percentage of poor and near-poor elderly was 38 percent compared with 22 percent for the total population. In 1983 the proportion had declined to 30.2 percent compared with 25.6 percent for the population as a whole. The percentage of the total "poverty population" who were aged 65 and over has declined in recent years, not because of a drop in the numbers of elderly poor but because of a large increase in the numbers of younger individuals in poverty.[10]

Almost 3.8 million elderly persons had incomes below the poverty threshold in 1982.[8] The highest poverty rates are among aged women, blacks, those who live alone, those who are not married, those who do not work, those who live in small towns and rural areas, and those who depend exclusively on Social Security benefits.[1] It was estimated, however, that without the transfer payments made under the Social Security system, 55 percent of the total elderly population would have been in poverty in 1982.[11]

Table 3-2. Median income of aged units* by age, sex and marital status, 1980 and 1982.

	Age group					
	55-61	62-64	65-67	68-72	73-79	80 & over
1980						
All units	16,880	12,800	9,780	7,810	6,650	4,820
Married couples	23,810	18,380	14,800	12,300	10,860	9,330
Nonmarried persons	7,910	6,330	5,510	5,240	4,830	4,210
Men	10,320	7,270	6,310	5,720	5,520	4,990
Women	7,110	5,970	5,250	5,130	4,710	4,040
1982						
All units	19,920	14,430	12,380	10,280	7,970	6,170
Married couples	26,250	20,370	17,930	16,210	13,900	11,070
Nonmarried persons	9,000	7,970	6,920	6,410	5,740	5,360
Men	11,780	10,690	8,840	7,400	7,160	6,250
Women	8,120	7,400	6,210	6,150	5,530	5,180

* An aged unit is a married couple living together or a nonmarried person.

Source: U.S. Department of Health and Human Services. Income of the population 55 and over, 1980. SSA Publication No. 13-11871, Social Security Administration, Office of Policy, Office of Research and Statistics. U.S. Government Printing Office, January 1983, and U.S. Department of Health and Human Services. Income of the population 55 and over, 1982. SSA Publication No. 13-11871, Social Security Administration Office of Policy, Office of Research and Statistics. U.S. Government Printing Office, March 1984.

Table 3-3. Income distribution of the total white and black populations and of those aged 55 and over, 1979.

Numbers in thousands

Age groups

White population:	Total all ages	55-64	65-74	75 & over
Population with income	147,187	18,501	14,748	8,269
Income: Less than $2,000	20,740	1,851	1,706	946
$2,000 to $5,000	37,913	4,526	6,414	4,489
$6,000 to $9,999	26,772	3,151	3,056	1,498
$10,000 to $24,999	48,805	6,853	2,762	1,090
$25,000 and over	12,958	2,472	657	246

Percentage

Population with income	100.0	100.0	100.0	100.0
Income: Less than $2,000	14.0	10.0	12.0	11.0
$2,000 to $5,000	26.0	24.0	43.0	54.0
$6,000 to $9,999	18.0	17.0	21.0	18.0
$10,000 to $24,999	33.0	37.0	19.0	13.0
$25,000 and over	9.0	13.0	4.0	3.0

Black population:				
Population with income;	15,224	1,669	1,245	680
Income: Less than $2,000	2,732	249	211	131
$2,000 to $5,999	4,908	598	746	465
$6,000 to $9,999	3,066	316	176	61
$10,000 to 24,999	3,991	448	101	22
$25,000 and Over	428	58	11	2

Percentage

Population with income:	100.0	100.0	100.0	100.0
Income: Less than $2,000	18.0	15.0	17.0	19.0
$2,000 to $5,999	32.0	36.0	60.0	68.0
$6,000 to $9,999	20.0	19.0	14.0	9.0
$10,000 to 24,999	26.0	27.0	8.0	3.0
$25,000 and Over	3.0	3.0	1.0	0.3

Source: U.S. Bureau of the Census: Census of the Population, 1980 Detailed Population Characteristics, United States Summary, PC80-1-D1-A. Washington, D.C., U.S. Government Printing Office, March 1984.

Table 3-6 shows the poverty rates for selected elderly subgroups in 1982, demonstrating that poverty rates have continued to decline but that those who belong to two or more of the subgroups at high risk of poverty have much higher rates. Whereas 15 percent of the total elderly population was living below the poverty line, 60 percent of elderly black women living alone were in poverty compared with 18 percent of all elderly

Table 3-4. Income distribution of the total male and female populations and of those aged 55 and over, 1979.

Numbers in thousands

Age groups

Male population:	Total all ages	55-64	65-74	75 & over
Population with income:	77,297	9,975	6,601	3,370
Income: Less than $2,000	6,788	366	242	215
$2,000 to $5,999	13,547	1,322	2,170	1,582
$6,000 to $9,999	11,992	1,370	2,119	795
$10,000 to $24,999	33,209	4,680	1,927	616
$25,000 and over	11,761	2,236	540	162

Percentage

Population with income:	100.0	100.0	100.0	100.0
Income: Less than $2,000	9.0	4.0	4.0	6.0
$2,000 to $5,999	18.0	13.0	33.0	47.0
$6,000 to $9,999	16.0	14.0	32.0	24.0
$10,000 to $24,999	43.0	47.0	29.0	18.0
$25,000 and over	15.0	22.0	8.0	5.0

Female population:	91,483	11,594	8,850	6,386
Population with income:	69,889	8,526	8,147	5,734
Income: Less than $2,000	13,952	1,485	1,464	887
$2,000 to $5,999	24,367	2,852	4,245	3,473
$6,000 to $9,999	14,778	1,781	1,334	781
$10,000 to $24,999	15,597	2,173	970	506
$25,000 and over	1,195	235	134	88

Percentage

Population with income:	100.0	100.0	100.0	100.0
Income: Less than $2,000	20.0	17.0	18.0	15.0
$2,000 to $5,999	35.0	33.0	52.0	61.0
$6,000 to $9,999	21.0	21.0	16.0	14.0
$10,000 to $24,999	22.0	25.0	12.0	9.0
$25,000 and over	2.0	3.0	2.0	2.0

Source: U.S. Bureau of the Census: Census of the Population, 1980. Detailed Population Characteristics, United States Summary, PC80-1-D1-A. Washington, D.C., U.S. Government Printing Office, March 1984.

women and 28 percent of all elderly living alone. The median income of black females is still well below the poverty line.

Means-Tested Benefits

SSI payments and other benefits are designed to provide assistance to the poor, but maximum federal benefits are set below the poverty level, which was defined as $4,626 for a married couple in 1982.[2]

Table 3-5. Median income for households with the householder aged 65 or over, by race and by state, 1979.

State	White Median income	Rank	Black Median income	Rank
United States*	$12,671		$9,356	
Alabama	9,810	48	6,927	37
Alaska	20,373	2	**	**
Arizona	13,176	14	8,670	27
Arkansas	9,409	51	6,091	40
California	14,682	8	9,878	19
Colorado	12,904	17	10,421	11
Connecticut	15,450	5	10,861	6
Delaware	13,833	11	9,656	23
District of Columbia	30,396	1	13,711	1
Florida	13,098	16	7,381	32
Georgia	11,178	40	7,109	36
Hawaii	20,099	3	**	**
Idaho	10,999	41	**	**
Illinois	14,830	7	10,610	9
Indiana	12,493	22	9,866	20
Iowa	12,628	21	10,234	14
Kansas	12,256	26	9,547	24
Kentucky	9,685	49	7,820	29
Louisiana	11,334	38	6,904	38
Maine	10,449	45	**	**
Maryland	15,728	4	10,151	16
Massachusetts	13,641	12	11,195	5
Michigan	12,322	25	10,376	12
Minnesota	11,687	33	10,597	10
Mississippi	9,450	50	6,272	39
Missouri	11,410	37	9,264	25
Montana	11,290	39	**	**
Nebraska	12,056	28	9,732	22
Nevada	14,208	9	11,474	4
New Hampshire	12,367	23	**	**
New Jersey	14,979	6	10,719	8
New Mexico	11,412	36	8,333	28
New York	14,194	10	10,368	13
North Carolina	10,937	42	7,694	30
North Dakota	11,499	35	**	**
Ohio	12,732	19	9,941	17
Oklahoma	10,470	44	7,458	31
Oregon	12,183	27	10,221	15
Pennsylvania	12,704	20	9,897	18
Rhode Island	12,352	24	12,197	2
South Carolina	11,617	34	7,113	35
South Dakota	9,958	47	**	**
Tennessee	10,113	46	7,369	33
Texas	12,047	29	7,283	34
Utah	12,752	18	**	**
Vermont	11,726	32	**	**
Virginia	13,288	13	8,822	26
Washington	13,146	15	11,503	3
West Virginia	10,609	43	9,790	21
Wisconsin	12,021	31	10,784	7
Wyoming	12,041	30	**	**

* Mean of medians does not include black income for deleted (**) states.

** Less than 500 persons of age and race in state.

Source: U.S. Bureau of the Census, Census of the Population, 1980. General Social and Economic Characteristics, United States Summary, PC80-1-C1. Washington, D.C., U.S. Government Printing Office, 1984.

Table 3-6. Poverty rates for selected elderly subgroups, 1982.

Elderly subgroup	Percentage below the poverty level
All elderly	15
Elderly women	18
Elderly living alone	28
Elderly blacks	42
Elderly black women living alone	66

Source: Tomorrow's elderly: issues for Congress. Report prepared for the House Select Committee on Aging by the Congressional Clearinghouse on the Future, 1984. Comm. Pub. No. 98-457. Washington, D.C., U.S. Government Printing Office, 1984.

Table 3-7 shows the maximum potential dollar value of SSI and food stamp benefits for the elderly by state in 1984. The maximum monthly federal benefit levels were $314 for a single person and $472 for married couples.[5] For individuals, the highest potential benefit values are in Alaska, Connecticut, and California. Some states appear to have higher supplementation rates for married couples than for individuals, notably California and Colorado. Approximately 40 percent of all SSI recipients receive a state supplement.[1]

It has been estimated by the Social Security Administration that only 65 to 70 percent of those aged 65 and over who are eligible for SSI actually take advantage of the program, and that 49 percent of elderly individuals living in poverty receive no cash or in-kind assistance from means-tested programs.[1]

The SSI program was established under the auspices of the federal government to help eradicate the "welfare" stigma.[1] The low participation rate by potential beneficiaries may indicate reluctance to be subjected to means testing or to lack of information regarding the program. While not statistically significant, the highest participation rates are in states providing supplements to federal payments, with no previous lien laws on the property of assistance recipients.[1]

The asset limitations of $1,500 for individuals and $2,250 for married couples also contribute to low enrollment of elderly and disabled individuals who would otherwise qualify for SSI on the basis of their incomes. It was estimated in 1983 that if the asset limits had been tied to the CPI, they would have increased by over 100 percent since the program began in 1974.[10]

Labor Force Participation

Table 3-8 demonstrates that labor force participation rates decline with advancing age for older persons, black and white, male and female. In 1981, at age 70, only 13 percent of men and 5 percent of women were working compared with 81 percent of men and 50 percent of women in the age group 55 to 59.

Table 3-7. Maximum potential dollar value of Supplemental Security Income and food stamp benefits for aged individuals, by state, January 1984

State	Combined benefits for individuals living independently		Combined benefits for couples living independently	
	Monthly	Annual	Monthly	Annual
Alabama	361.00	4332.00	535.00	6420.00
Alaska	621.00	7452.00	897.00	10764.00
Arizona	361.00	4332.00	535.00	6420.00
Arkansas	361.00	4332.00	535.00	6420.00
California	477.00	5724.00	886.00	10632.00
Colorado	402.00	4824.00	754.00	9048.00
Connecticut	490.30	5883.60	770.60	9247.20
Delaware	361.00	4332.00	535.00	6420.00
District of Columbia	372.00	4464.00	556.00	6672.00
Florida	361.00	4332.00	535.00	6420.00
Georgia	361.00	4332.00	535.00	6420.00
Hawaii	423.90	5086.80	627.80	7533.60
Idaho	423.00	5076.00	576.00	6912.00
Illinois	361.00	4332.00	550.45	6605.40
Indiana	361.00	4332.00	535.00	6420.00
Iowa	361.00	4332.00	535.00	6420.00
Kansas	361.00	4332.00	535.00	6420.00
Kentucky	361.00	4332.00	535.00	6420.00
Louisiana	361.00	4332.00	535.00	6420.00
Maine	368.00	4416.00	545.00	6540.00
Maryland	361.00	4332.00	535.00	6420.00
Massachusetts	452.00	5424.00	683.72	8204.64
Michigan	378.30	4539.60	560.40	6724.80
Minnesota	386.00	4632.00	581.00	6972.00
Mississippi	361.00	4332.00	535.00	6420.00
Missouri	361.00	4332.00	535.00	6420.00
Montana	361.00	4332.00	535.00	6420.00
Nebraska	413.50	4962.00	610.50	7326.00
Nevada	386.40	4636.80	587.46	7049.52
New Hampshire	380.00	4560.00	550.00	6600.00
New Jersey	387.17	4646.04	556.28	6675.36
New Mexico	361.00	4332.00	535.00	6420.00
New York	403.91	4846.92	588.03	7056.36
North Carolina	361.00	4332.00	535.00	6420.00
North Dakota	361.00	4332.00	535.00	6420.00
Ohio	361.00	4332.00	535.00	6420.00
Oklahoma	410.00	4920.00	636.00	7632.00
Oregon	362.70	4352.40	535.00	6420.00
Pennsylvania	384.40	4612.80	568.70	6824.40
Rhode Island	397.98	4775.76	603.30	7239.60
South Carolina	361.00	4332.00	535.00	6420.00
South Dakota	372.00	4464.00	545.00	6540.00
Tennessee	361.00	4332.00	535.00	6420.00
Texas	361.00	4332.00	535.00	6420.00
Utah	368.00	4416.00	549.00	6588.00
Vermont	396.00	4752.00	599.00	7188.00
Virginia	361.00	4332.00	535.00	6420.00
Washington	388.30	4659.60	560.40	6724.80
West Virginia	361.00	4332.00	535.00	6420.00
Wisconsin	413.70	4964.40	633.00	7596.00
Wyoming	375.00	4500.00	563.00	6756.00

Source: Special Committee on Aging, U.S. Senate. The proposed fiscal year 1984 budget: what it means for older Americans. Washington, D.C., U.S. Government Printing Office, 1983.

Table 3-8. Labor force participation ratios for the population 55 years and over, by age, race and sex, selected years 1955-1981.

			Year			
All races	1955	1960	1965	1970	1975	1981
Males aged:						
55 to 64	87.9	86.8	84.7	83.0	75.8	70.8
55 to 59	92.5	91.6	90.2	89.5	84.4	81.3
60 to 64	82.5	81.2	78.0	75.0	65.7	58.7
65 years & over	39.6	33.1	27.9	26.8	21.7	18.5
65 to 69	57.0	46.8	43.0	41.6	31.7	27.8
70 years & over	28.1	24.4	19.1	17.7	15.1	12.6
Females aged:						
55 to 64	32.5	37.2	41.1	43.0	41.0	41.5
55 to 59	35.6	42.2	47.1	49.0	47.9	49.9
60 to 64	29.0	31.4	34.0	36.1	33.3	32.7
65 years & over	10.6	10.8	10.0	9.7	8.3	8.1
65 to 69	17.8	17.6	17.4	17.3	14.5	14.9
70 years & over	6.4	6.8	6.1	5.7	4.9	4.6
Black and other races						
Males aged:						
55 to 64	83.1	82.5	78.8	79.2	68.7	63.2
55 to 59	NA	NA	NA	83.5	76.9	72.0
60 to 64	NA	NA	NA	73.6	59.3	52.6
65 years & over	40.0	31.2	27.9	27.4	20.9	16.8
Females aged:						
55 to 64	40.7	47.3	48.9	47.1	43.8	44.9
55 to 59	NA	NA	NA	53.4	52.1	50.8
60 to 64	NA	NA	NA	39.0	34.6	37.9
65 years & over	12.1	12.8	12.9	12.2	10.5	9.3

NA: Not available

Source: U.S. Bureau of the Census, Current Population Reports, Series P-23, No. 138, Demographic and socioeconomic aspects of aging in the United States. Washington, D.C., U.S. Government Printing Office, 1984.

Of greater significance is the progressive decline in the proportion of men in the labor force (i.e., working or looking for work) at older ages. Ninety-two percent of men aged 55 to 59 were working in 1960 compared with 81 percent in 1981. The trend for elderly black men has been the same as for white men, although the participation rate at all ages is lower for black men than white men.

In contrast, there has been an increase in the proportion of older women in the labor force during the past thirty years, with 50 percent of women aged 55 to 59 years working in 1981 compared with 36 percent in 1955; although the trend in labor force participation for black women has been the same as for white women, the percentage working at older ages is higher for black women than for white.

A number of factors have been proposed to account for the lower labor force participation of older men, including: voluntary retirement associated with more widespread eligibility for Social Security and other pension plans; the decline in self-employment; and discrimination against older workers and pressures exerted by employers on older workers to retire.[9] Increasing the age of eligibility for social insurance payments or failure to index benefits to the CPI would lead many elderly persons to seek to remain in the work force to more advanced ages.

Economic Dependency Ratios

Table 3-9 shows the total population by age group, with dependency ratios for the aged and for the whole population, from 1960 to 1980, with

Table 3-9. Social Security population and dependency ratios by broad age group, 1960-2060.

| | Population in thousands | | | | Dependency ratio | |
Calendar year	Under 20	20-64	65 & over	Total	Aged *	Total **
1960	73,108	98,689	17,147	188,943	0.174	0.915
1965	79,959	104,121	18,952	203,032	0.182	0.950
1970	80,737	112,606	20,681	214,024	0.184	0.901
1975	79,041	122,615	23,300	224,956	0.190	0.835
1980	75,620	134,475	26,321	236,417	0.196	0.758
Projections ***						
1985	73,811	144,510	29,406	247,727	0.203	0.714
1990	74,747	151,265	32,659	258,670	0.216	0.710
1995	76,336	157,178	35,077	268,590	0.223	0.709
2000	77,192	163,823	36,338	277,353	0.222	0.693
2005	76,486	171,436	37,681	285,603	0.220	0.666
2010	76,311	176,767	40,687	293,765	0.230	0.662
2015	77,108	177,840	46,492	301,440	0.261	0.695
2020	78,325	176,605	53,222	308,152	0.301	0.745
2025	79,097	174,079	60,584	313,759	0.348	0.802
2030	79,257	172,948	66,215	318,420	0.383	0.841
2035	79,410	174,193	68,673	322,275	0.394	0.850
2040	79,937	176,402	69,014	325,354	0.391	0.844
2045	80,711	178,177	68,860	327,748	0.386	0.839
2050	81,381	178,466	69,919	329,766	0.392	0.848
2055	81,817	178,929	71,100	331,846	0.397	0.855
2060	82,179	180,213	71,913	334,305	0.399	0.855

*Population aged 65 and over as ratio to the population aged 20 to 64.

**Population aged 65 and over plus population under age 20 as ratio to the population aged 20 to 64.

*** Assuming fertility rates of 2.0 children per woman and reductions in mortality at an average annual rate of 0.6 percent per year from 1981-2057.

Source: Annual Report - Federal Old-Age and Survivors Insurance and and Disability Insurance Trust Fund, 1983. House Document No. 98-74. Washington, D.C., U.S. Government Printing Office, 1984.

middle-series projections from 1985 to 2060. The aged dependency ratio has increased from 0.174 to 0.203 between 1960 and 1985 and is projected to remain at less than 0.3 until after 2015. The total dependency ratio, which includes those under age 20, together with the elderly, has led to an overall decline in the rate since 1960 because of lower birthrates. Assuming fertility rates of 2.0 children per woman, the total dependency ratio is projected to decline continuously to 2010. An increase in fertility rates would therefore increase the dependency ratio in the immediate future but would then lead to a decline when these individuals entered the work force.

Social Security Program: Future Trends

The Social Security program is affected by many factors, including increasing life expectancy, labor force participation rates, and the overall level of economic activity. When the 1972 amendments to the Social Security Act increased benefits across the board by 20 percent and initiated indexing, future projections were for continuing relatively high economic growth and low rates of inflation.[1] Since that time, growth rates have not been sustained, and there have been periods of high inflation, recession, and unemployment. Indexing benefits caused major increases in expenditures during the period of high inflation, while unemployment and low growth in real wages lowered the payroll tax income to the OASDI funds. In addition to the recent economic changes, declining mortality rates for the very elderly since 1970 have increased projections of the number of beneficiaries.

Table 3-10 shows a comparison between the number of OASDI beneficiaries and the number of covered workers between 1945 and 1982, with projections to the year 2050. In 1945 there were only two beneficiaries per 100 covered workers and 42 covered workers per OASDI beneficiary. By 1981 this had increased to 31 beneficiaries per 100 workers and 3.2 workers per beneficiary. These ratios are predicted to remain relatively constant until 2015, when the number of beneficiaries will begin to increase and there will be a commensurate decline in the proportion of covered workers.

Predictions regarding the relationship between contributions and benefits for the maintenance of the Social Security program between now and the middle of the next century vary. The 1983 amendments to the Social Security Act, which included incentives to defer retirement and a gradual increase in the retirement age after the year 2000, were designed to maintain the OASDI funds for the first quarter of the next century. An increase in the birthrate, combined with sustained economic growth, would insure the continuing financial stability of the program.

Table 3-10. Comparison of OASDI beneficiaries and covered workers, 1945-2060.

Calendar year	Covered workers (thousands)	Beneficiaries (thousands)	Covered workers per OASDI beneficiary
1945	46,390	1,106	41.9
1950	48,280	2,930	16.5
1955	65,200	7,563	8.6
1960	72,530	14,262	5.1
1965	80,680	20,157	4.0
1970	93,090	25,186	3.7
1975	100,200	31,123	3.2
1980	114,300	35,119	3.3
1981	115,800	35,710	3.2
1982	115,000	35,391	3.2
Projections:			
1983	115,220	35,811	3.2
1985	123,865	36,995	3.3
1990	134,485	40,452	3.3
1995	141,308	42,933	3.3
2000	147,917	44,699	3.3
2005	153,326	47,498	3.2
2010	156,199	51,067	3.1
2015	156,831	57,224	2.7
2020	156,612	64,040	2.4
2025	156,727	70,512	2.2
2030	157,341	75,027	2.1
2035	158,234	77,533	2.0
2040	159,006	78,110	2.0
2045	159,717	78,683	2.0
2050	160,588	79,661	2.0

Source: Annual Report - Federal Old-Age and Survivors Insurance and Disability Insurance Trust Fund, 1983. House Document No. 98-74. Washington, D.C., U.S. Government Printing Office, 1984.

Summary

Over the past twenty-five years the income of the elderly has been increasing and poverty rates have declined at a faster rate than for other sectors of the population. The Social Security system, through the benefits provided under the OASDI program, has been a major factor in contributing to the improved financial status of the elderly. Without these transfer payments and the income protection provided by Medicare against health care costs, poverty rates would be substantially higher.

On the other hand, there is still wide variation in income distribution by state, sex, race, marital status, and age group and income declines with age for all elderly subgroups. Women, blacks, and the very aged have higher-than-average poverty rates among the elderly, but there is low uptake of means-tested benefits by those with incomes below the poverty line who are potentially eligible for SSI payments and food stamps.

Although there has been a small increase in elderly female labor force participation, there has been a decline in the proportion of elderly men in the work force, with an increase in the percentage receiving reduced retirement benefits at earlier ages.

Over the next thirty years the number of beneficiaries to workers will increase, causing potential problems in funding OASDI benefits, particularly if the existing trends to early retirement continue. Recent amendments have been introduced to ensure the solvency of the fund until after the year 2020. These include financial incentives to defer the age of retirement and a gradual increase in the age at which full Social Security benefits are payable, from 65 to 67 years.

More increases in the age at which workers become eligible for Social Security benefits, increasing payroll contributions, and taxing benefits and withholding them from those with other sources of income have all been proposed as measures to maintain the OASDI funds as the beneficiary-to-worker ratio increases in the next 50 years.

The extent to which older workers are able to defer retirement will depend on individual health status, the extent to which there is competition with younger workers, and overall economic activity rates. Sustained economic growth and low inflation, combined with an increase in the birthrate, could avert any future crisis in funding Social Security entitlements and improve the projected worker-to-beneficiary ratios.

REFERENCES

1. Developments in aging: Vol. 1, 1982. A report of the Special Committee on Aging, United States Senate. Washington, D.C. U.S. Government Printing Office, 1983.
2. Tomorrow's elderly: issues for Congress. Report prepared for the House Select Committee on Aging by the Congressional Clearinghouse on the Future, 1984. Comm. Pub. No. 98-457, Washington, D.C. U.S. Government Printing Office, 1984.
3. Torrey B. B. Sharing increasing costs on declining income: the visible dilemma of the invisible aged. Milbank Memorial Fund Quarterly 63: 377–394, Spring, 1985.
4. Annual Report—Federal Old-Age and Survivors Insurance and Disability Insurance Trust Fund, 1983. House Document No. 98-74, Washington, D.C. U.S. Government Printing Office, 1984.
5. Background data on programs within the jurisdiction of the Committee on Ways and Means, House of Representatives Washington, D.C. U.S. Government Printing Office, 1984.
6. The Supplemental Security Income Program for the aged, blind and disabled: selected characteristics of State Supplementation Programs as of January

1984. SSA Pub. No. 13-11975, U.S. Department of Health and Human Services. U.S. Government Printing Office, December, 1984.

7. U.S. Department of Health and Human Services. Income of the population 55 and over, 1980. SSA Pub. No. 13-11871, Social Security Administration, Office of Policy, Office of Research and Statistics. U.S. Government Printing Office, January 1983.

8. U.S. Department of Health and Human Services. Income of the Population 55 and Over, 1982. SSA Pub. No. 13-11871, Social Security Administration, Office of Policy, Office of Research and Statistics. U.S. Government Printing Office, March 1984.

9. U.S. Bureau of the Census, Current Population Reports, Series P-23, No. 138, Demographic and socioeconomic aspects of aging in the United States. Washington, D.C. U.S. Government Printing Office, 1984.

10. Penner R. G., Director, Congressional Budget Office. Statement before the Subcommittee on Oversight and the Subcommittee on Public Assistance and Unemployment Compensation, Ways and Means Committee, U.S. House of Representatives, October 18, 1983.

11. Stockman D. A., Director, Office of Management and Budget. Testimony to the House Committee on Ways and Means, Subcommittee on Oversight and Subcommittee on Public Assistance and Unemployment Compensation. 98th Congress, 1st Session, November 3, 1983. Washington, D.C. U.S. Government Printing Office, 1983.

4

Mortality, Morbidity, and Functional Disability

Mortality rates have declined, with consequent increases in life expectancy, throughout the 20th century. In the early decades improvements were concentrated among younger age groups. In the 1940's and 1950's substantial mortality declines continued, with the changes spread more evenly across the age spectrum. From 1955 to 1967 mortality rates remained relatively constant; in recent years the downward trend has resumed for all age groups, including the extreme elderly.[1-4]

The reasons for mortality decline, the likelihood of a continuing linear trend as opposed to a cyclical pattern of mortality reductions, and the outcome in terms of prevalence of chronic disease morbidity and functional disability are all subject to debate.[5-10] From the late 19th century, falling mortality rates have resulted from public health measures, better nutrition, and control of infectious disease. In recent years prevention or control of chronic disease processes seems to account for increased life expectancy among older age groups.

In 1980 Fries argued that life expectancy increases had occurred as a result of the progressive elimination of "premature death" in the young, but that the maximum life span of the human race had not increased.[5] Citing evidence from experimental studies of cellular senescence, Fries proposed 85 years as the age of "natural death" for human beings. As life expectancy increases toward this age, survival rates between birth and death may be plotted as a progressively more rectangular curve, with individuals surviving from birth to old age and then dying within a relatively short time period. Fries further argued that variation between individuals in functional ability at all ages demonstrates that it should be possible to postpone the onset of chronic disease morbidity and maintain vigor until near the end of this fixed life span. These theories have been widely disputed.[6-10]

Analysis of the recent decline in mortality rates for those aged 85 and over, and confident predictions that this trend will continue, refute the concept of "rectangularization of the survival curve."[6,7] While an alternative natural life span of 100 years has also been proposed, even the number of centenarians has shown a marked increase.[4]

52

Others have challenged Fries' theories of "natural death" and "compression of morbidity," arguing that no mortality occurs in the absence of disease and expressing concern at the possible effects that the acceptance of such optimistic theories would have on health care planning and policy for the elderly.[6-8] Some argue that recent increases in life expectancy represent the "failures of success." Advances in medical technology have been instrumental in arresting the once-fatal complications of disease processes; this has resulted in an increased life expectancy for the sick and disabled, with a "rising pandemic" of chronic disease, mental disorders, and associated disabilities.[9,10]

The relationship between declining mortality and morbidity and between morbidity and prevalence rates of functional disability have important implications for projecting the future need for medical and other long-term care services.

Self-reported morbidity for middle-aged and older people increased between 1957 and 1979,[11] while a study of data for 1966 to 1976 found an increase in morbidity and associated disability rates for all age groups, not just the elderly.[12] A number of reasons may account for this apparent increase, including earlier diagnosis, willingness to adopt the "sick role," and improved survival rates for acute episodes of illness.[11] If disease incidence is constant or increasing, mortality reductions will result in higher prevalence and duration of disease. On the other hand, the progression of disease processes may be retarded by health-promoting activities or medical intervention.

From 1950 to 1978 the incidence of heart disease was virtually unchanged and the incidence of cancer increased, yet the age at death for individuals dying of these conditions also increased. The increase in the age of death for women dying of heart disease or cancer was, however, much greater than for men.[7] Although mortality rates have declined constantly over time for both sexes, mortality differences between elderly men and women have increased. In 1940 the age-adjusted death rate for males was 22 percent higher than for females, and in 1978 it was 73 percent higher.[1]

Progress in controlling risk factors such as diet, cigarette smoking, and hypertension, as well as positive developments in the treatment and rehabilitation of patients with coronary heart disease and stroke, may all have contributed to the decline in mortality rates for older age groups. The implication is that further reductions, particularly in male mortality, are still possible, although there is also evidence that the innate hormonal differences between the sexes are instrumental in delaying the onset of cardiovascular disease in females.

For most chronic diseases, women have higher reported prevalence rates than men.[11] On the other hand, the higher disease-specific mortality rates of elderly men compared with women for most leading causes of death indicate either that the diseases common to older men tend to be more life threatening than those prevalent among older women or that the rate of progression in the diseases with high associated morbidity is slower in women than in men. An alternative explanation is that there are higher rates of disease diagnosis in women, associated with higher physician consultation rates for women than men.[13]

Osteoporotic and arthritic conditions undoubtedly have higher prevalence rates among elderly women than men and, together with their longer life expectancy, lead to a higher probability of elderly women suffering long-term functional disability. As with the complex relationship between mortality and morbidity, however, there is no clear association between morbidity and functional disability.

Until recent years, surveys treated those aged 65 and over as a homogeneous group, but age-specific and activity-specific data now demonstrate that morbidity, disability, and dependency rates increase substantially with each advancing age cohort, both among the institutionalized and those living in the community. Women consistently show higher disability rates than men, as do blacks compared with whites and the poor compared with higher-income groups.[14–19] On the other hand, the elderly encompass a thirty-five year age range and, although most elderly individuals report symptoms of at least one chronic disease, the majority of individuals do not suffer from functional disability or need assistance, even in the oldest age groups.

In view of the fact that national surveys to determine prevalence estimates for functional disability have only recently been undertaken, there are no time series data to compare the levels of morbidity and functional impairment in the present elderly generation with those of the past. It is therefore not known if those who are now living to advanced old age suffer higher levels of chronic morbidity and related functional disability than the much smaller proportion of individuals who showed great longevity twenty or forty years ago. Nor are data available on the characteristics or lifestyle of those who survive into advanced old age without any physical or mental impairment.

The concept of the "compression of morbidity" suggests an idealistic goal that might eventually be achieved with a major allocation of resources to health education and preventive medicine for the young. All recent demographic, mortality, and morbidity data, however, support those who predict a major increase, if not a "pandemic," of individuals afflicted with chronic degenerative disease well into the next century and a commensurate growth in the number who are functionally disabled.

DATA SOURCES

Sources of information for the tables presented in this chapter are as follows.

Data on national mortality for all certified deaths are collected continuously and made available by the National Center for Health Statistics (NCHS).[1-3]

Morbidity and functional disability data are based on estimates from sample surveys. The NCHS conducts periodic surveys of the characteristics of the nursing home population, including morbidity and disability levels.[14] The latest survey is being conducted in 1985. The NCHS also provides data from the National Health Interview Survey. This has a multistage design that permits continuous sampling of the noninstitutionalized population. In 1979 and 1980 a Home Care Supplement was included, from which data have been analyzed and published.[15,16]

The 1982 National Long-Term Care Survey of the noninstitutionalized population aged 65 and over was conducted under the sponsorship of the Health Care Financing Administration and other agencies of the Department of Health and Human Services. Functionally disabled elderly persons living in the community, and their primary caregivers, were interviewed following screening of a random sample of all elderly Medicare enrollees. Some data from this survey have now become available, while others currently are being analyzed.[17-19] A follow-up survey of the same population was conducted in 1984.

Prevalence estimates of psychiatric morbidity are available from the National Institute of Mental Health multisite program and from other recent community surveys.[19-22]

Mortality

Age Group Differences

Table 4-1, computed from national statistics, shows mortality rates of age groups 65 and over for the years 1950, 1960, 1970, 1980, 1983, and the percentage change over time. The overall rate of decline was 31 percent for those aged 75 to 84, 27 percent for the age group 65 to 74, and 22 percent for those aged 85 and over.

Official data show that the rate of decline was higher for the 85 and over age group than for other adult cohorts from the middle 1960's to the middle 1970's. Medicare enrollment data were used to test the accuracy of population estimates for the extreme aged used in reporting official mortality statistics between 1966 and 1977. These confirmed a substantial real reduction in mortality for this age group but, even though the rate of decline for the extreme aged was no higher than for a number of other age groups, the rate of change did exceed that of previous decades.[2]

Table 4-2 gives the age-adjusted and age-specific death rates for the leading causes of death for the total population and for age groups 55 and over for the years 1979, 1981, and 1982. This shows a fluctuation in mortality rates for those aged 85 and over but a steady decline for other older

Table 4-1. Death rates of the population aged 65 and over, by age group, and percentage change over time, 1950, 1960, 1970, 1980 and 1983.

Rate per 100,000

Age group	1950	1960	1970	1980	1983
65-74	4067.7	3822.1	3582.7	2994.9	2883.4
75-84	9331.1	8745.2	8004.4	6692.6	6309.7
85 & over	20196.9	19857.5	17539.4	15980.3	15422.3

Percentage change

Age group	1950-60	1960-70	1970-80	1980-83	Overall change
65-74	-4.56	-6.26	-16.41	-3.72	-30.95
75-84	-6.28	-8.47	-16.39	-5.72	-36.86
85 & over	-1.68	-11.67	-8.88	-2.87	-25.10

Source: National Center for Health Statistics: Health, United States, 1984. DHHS Publication No. (PHS)85-1232, Public Health Service. Washington, D.C. U.S. Government Printing Office, December 1984.

age groups, thus ensuring a continuing growth in the number of very elderly in the population.

Disease-Specific Causes

Disease-specific mortality rates, as shown in Table 4-2, demonstrate that three leading causes of death—heart disease, cerebrovascular disease, and cancer—account for three quarters of all deaths of individuals aged 65 and over, with heart disease accounting for nearly one half the total. Reductions in the risk of dying from the first two declined substantially from the middle 1960's to the 1970's for all age groups, including those aged 85 and over.[2] Table 4-2 indicates a continued decline in mortality from cerebrovascular disease for all older age groups between 1979 and 1982 and from heart disease for all except those aged 85 and over. Death rates for pneumonia and influenza fluctuate from year to year; deaths from renal disorders and septicemia, which contribute little to overall rates, have shown a small progressive increase for all older age groups.

Male-Female Ratios

In spite of decreasing mortality rates for both sexes, mortality differences between men and women aged 65 and over have increased steadily

Table 4-2. Age-specific and age-adjusted death rates for 10 leading causes, 1979, 1981 and 82.

Cause of death (Ninth Revision International Classification of Diseases, 1975)	Year	All ages	55-64	65-74	75-84	85 & over	Age-adjusted rate
All causes	1982	852.0	1297.9	2885.2	6329.8	15048.3	553.8
	1981	862.4	1322.1	2922.3	6429.9	15379.7	568.2
	1979	852.2	1338.0	2929.0	6496.6	14962.4	577.0
Diseases of heart 390-398,402,404-429	1982	326.0	468.7	1156.4	2801.4	7341.8	190.5
	1981	328.7	481.5	1175.8	2850.3	7458.8	195.0
	1979	326.5	499.0	1199.8	2925.2	7310.9	199.5
All forms of cancer 140-208	1982	187.2	439.7	824.9	1238.7	1598.6	132.5
	1981	184.0	434.8	814.8	1221.8	1575.3	131.6
	1979	179.6	429.4	800.0	1207.6	1522.9	130.8
Cerebrovascular diseases......430-438	1982	68.0	58.9	193.5	675.1	2000.8	35.8
	1981	71.3	62.9	206.3	715.6	2126.8	38.1
	1979	75.5	68.1	226.9	793.8	2264.9	41.6
Accidents and adverse effects.....E800-E949	1982	40.6	37.3	50.9	103.9	255.9	36.6
	1981	43.9	40.4	54.3	108.2	273.3	39.8
	1979	46.9	43.5	58.8	117.8	276.0	42.9
Chronic obstructive pulmonary diseases and allied conditions....490-496	1982	25.8	41.7	131.2	236.0	278.0	16.2
	1981	25.7	43.3	132.6	231.5	274.7	16.3
	1979	22.2	40.2	117.0	200.6	230.2	14.6
Pneumonia and influenza.....480-487	1982	21.1	16.4	47.6	183.4	747.8	10.9
	1981	23.4	18.4	52.5	209.3	845.8	12.3
	1979	20.1	16.4	47.8	184.2	694.9	11.2
Diabetes mellitus..250	1982	14.9	25.5	60.1	125.4	212.1	9.6
	1981	15.1	25.6	61.9	127.7	217.2	9.8
	1979	14.8	25.8	61.3	130.3	211.6	9.8
Atherosclerosis....440	1982	11.6	4.5	20.6	102.9	563.0	4.8
	1981	12.2	4.5	21.4	112.1	608.7	5.2
	1979	12.8	4.8	24.4	125.3	649.1	5.7
Nephritis, nephrotic syndrome, and nephrosis....580-589	1982	7.8	9.3	25.8	69.7	182.8	4.5
	1981	7.5	8.8	25.3	68.8	172.0	4.5
	1979	7.0	8.5	23.7	64.7	155.2	4.3
Septicemia..........038	1982	5.0	6.8	15.8	41.1	106.9	3.0
	1981	4.6	6.3	14.4	37.7	95.1	2.9
	1979	3.6	4.9	12.4	29.7	70.3	2.3

Source: National Center for Health Statistics: Advance report, final mortality statistics, 1982. Monthly Vital Statistics Report, Vol. 33, No. 9 Supp. DHHS Pub. No. (PHS)85-1120. Public Health Service, Hyattsville, Md., December 20, 1984.

Table 4-3. Ratio of male to female death rates for the ten leading causes of death for the population 65 years and over, by age, 1978.

Cause of death by rank *	65 & over	Age group 65-74	75-84	85 & over
All causes	1.450	1.958	1.601	1.275
1. Diseases of the heart	1.405	2.141	1.525	1.197
2. Malignant neoplasms	1.788	1.829	1.929	1.876
3. Cerebrovascular diseases	0.973	1.394	1.137	0.976
4. Influenza and pneumonia	1.487	2.263	1.890	1.521
5. Arteriosclerosis	0.923	1.609	1.218	1.035
6. Diabetes mellitus	0.875	0.998	0.915	0.917
7. Accidents	1.616	2.143	1.740	1.481
Motor vehicle	2.361	2.139	2.513	4.217
All other	1.434	2.145	1.551	1.336
8. Bronchitis, emphysema, and asthma	3.840	3.593	4.766	3.795
9. Cirrhosis of liver	2.579	2.589	2.300	2.339
10. Nephritis and nephrosis	1.685	1.653	2.019	1.967
All other causes	1.697	2.096	1.925	1.508

* Based on National Center for Health Statistics, Eighth Revision International Classification of Diseases, adapted for use in the United States, PHS Pub. No. 1693, 1967. The ten leading causes of death were defined on the basis of rates for the population 65 years and over for both sexes combined.

Source: U.S. Bureau of the Census, Current Population Reports, Series P-23, No. 138, Demographic and socioeconomic aspects of aging in the United States. Washington, D.C., U.S. Government Printing Office, 1984.

because of the very high rate of decrease in white female mortality.[1,2] Table 4-3 shows the ratio of male-to-female death rates for the ten leading causes of death for the population aged 65 and over in 1978.

Death rates for the two leading causes of death—diseases of the heart and malignant neoplasms—are much greater for males than females. Between 1950 and 1980, the mean age at death for women dying of heart disease rose by 5.44 years to age 82; for men it rose by only 2.75 years to age 75.[7] There is also considerable excess mortality for men from chronic lung diseases, cirrhosis of the liver, renal disease, and accidents. The only leading causes of death showing similar or slightly higher rates for women are cerebrovascular disease, arteriosclerosis, and diabetes.

Recent data have shown marginally higher rates of mortality decline for men than for women, although the age-adjusted death rate for males in 1982 was 1.8 times that for females.[3] It is predicted that differences in mortality rates and, consequently, in life expectancy will remain great in spite of some narrowing of differences.[4]

Racial Differences

Life expectancy at birth is some five years higher for whites than blacks but, at age 65, there is less than two years difference and at age 75 life expectancy is greater for blacks than for whites (11.2 years compared with 10.3 years in 1978).[4] As shown in Table 4-4, most of the difference between races is accounted for by the much lower mortality of whites at ages under 65, whereas at ages 80 to 84 mortality rates are lower for black than for white males and for those aged 85 and over mortality rates are lower for blacks of both sexes than for whites.

Table 4-5 shows the ratio of black to white mortality for ten leading causes of death in the population aged 65 and over in 1978. In the 65 to 74 age group, mortality rates were higher for blacks than whites for all leading causes of death except chronic lung disease and cirrhosis of the liver but, by age 85, rates were much lower for blacks for all causes except renal disease.

Chronic Disease Morbidity

Morbidity estimates must take account of those living in the community and of the institutionalized population. Data for the two populations are not necessarily comparable in that surveys of the noninstitutionalized population rely on self-reporting by individuals and their families, while morbidity rates among nursing home residents are based on clinical diagnoses.

Institutionalized Population

The primary diagnosis for 44 percent of the nursing home population aged 65 and over in 1977 was circulatory disease, with mental disorders forming the next-highest diagnostic category, at 16 percent. Other primary diagnoses among nursing home residents were diabetes in 6 percent, diseases of the musculoskeletal system, including arthritis, in 5 percent, and hip and other fractures in 3 percent.[14]

Noninstitutionalized Population

Eighty percent of the noninstitutionalized elderly report at least one chronic condition. As shown in Table 4-6, arthritis, hypertension, hearing loss, and heart disease account for 60 percent of these chronic conditions. There was a 125-percent increase in the percentage with heart conditions among those aged 65 and over compared with the population aged 45 to 64, a 55-percent increase in the percentage with hypertensive disease, and for hearing loss and visual impairments the increases were 100 percent and 147 percent, respectively. By contrast, there was only a 7-percent

Table 4-4. Deaths and death rates per 100,000 population in specified group, by age, race and sex, 1982.

Age	All races			White		
	Both sexes	Male	Female	Both sexes	Male	Female
			Number			
All ages	1,974,797	1,056,440	918,357	1,729,085	919,239	809,846
			Rate			
All ages*	852.0	938.0	770.7	872.9	951.8	797.9
Age 45-49	419.8	546.1	300.4	378.0	489.8	270.2
50-54	676.3	892.0	625.0	625.0	824.9	435.9
55-59	1039.2	1386.8	978.3	978.3	1308.7	680.0
60-64	1579.9	2123.5	1508.5	1508.5	2035.6	1050.5
65-69	2385.4	3256.1	2319.5	2319.5	3176.9	1624.5
70-74	3506.4	4817.6	3447.0	3447.0	4765.1	2494.1
75-79	5252.1	7183.2	5235.0	5235.0	7210.0	4006.1
80-84	8081.4	10582.7	8091.6	8091.6	10675.4	6752.7
85 & over	15048.3	17782.0	15296.9	15296.9	18123.1	14123.9

Age	Total			All other	Black	
	Both sexes	Male	Female	Both sexes	Male	Female
All ages						
				Number		
All ages	245,712	137,201	108,511	226,513	125,610	100,903
All ages*						
				Rate		
	728.9	854.8	614.5	819.2	960.4	692.4
Age 45-49	694.1	944.8	485.8	791.2	1093.4	545.7
50-54	1057.0	1433.3	754.4	1196.6	1630.8	848.9
55-59	1528.8	2054.9	1108.2	1717.4	2327.9	1233.6
60-64	2207.7	2934.7	1628.3	2446.1	3262.3	1805.5
65-69	2985.2	4001.1	2225.8	3269.0	4416.3	2429.6
70-74	4048.4	5295.0	3143.7	4386.3	5836.0	3385.1
75-79	5428.2	6935.4	4419.9	5791.8	7436.6	4726.4
80-84	7973.2	9786.1	6883.3	8532.5	10448.2	7417.1
85 & over	1259.6	14386.4	11130.5	12792.4	15117.9	11660.0

* Figures for "age not stated" included in "all ages" but not distributed among age groups.

Source: National Center for Health Statistics: Advance report, final mortality statistics, 1982. Monthly Vital Statistics Report, Vol.33, No.9 Supp. DHHS Pub.No.(PHS)85-1120, Public Health Service, Hyattsville, Md., December 1984.

Table 4-5. Ratio of black and other races to white death rates for the ten leading
causes of death for the population 65 years and over, by age, 1978

Cause of death by rank *	65 & over	65-74	75-84	85 & over
All causes	0.972	1.223	1.057	0.603
1. Diseases of the heart	0.862	1.100	0.954	0.547
2. Malignant neoplasms	1.021	1.120	1.061	0.694
3. Cerebrovascular diseases	1.096	1.836	1.193	0.599
4. Influenza and pneumonia	0.842	1.413	0.977	0.490
5. Arteriosclerosis	0.720	1.345	0.931	0.467
6. Diabetes mellitus	1.528	1.993	1.572	0.783
7. Accidents	1.050	1.423	1.092	0.555
Motor vehicle	1.083	1.160	1.133	0.685
All other	1.039	1.573	1.078	0.540
8. Bronchitis, emphysema, and asthma	0.457	0.481	0.470	0.411
9. Cirrhosis of liver	0.856	0.912	0.706	0.523
10. Nephritis and nephrosis	2.522	3.234	2.737	1.442
All other causes	1.163	1.345	1.250	0.844

* Based on National Center for Health Statistics, Eighth Revision International
Classification of Diseases, adapted for use in the United States, PHS Pub. No. 1693,
1967. The ten leading causes were defined on the basis of rates for the population 65
years and over for all races combined.

Source: U.S. Bureau of the Census, Current Population Reports, Series P-23, No.
138, Demographic and socioeconomic aspects of aging in the United States.
Washington, D.C., U.S. Government Printing Office, 1984.

increase in the proportion of the elderly reporting arthritis compared with
those aged 45 to 64.

Table 4-7 shows that elderly women have higher prevalence rates than
men for nearly all the leading chronic conditions, both those associated
with fatal complications such as hypertension, heart conditions, and arteriosclerosis and those associated with functional disability, such as arthritis and orthopedic impairments. The simple recording of disease prevalence does not indicate differences in disease severity between sexes or
age groups nor the level of any associated functional disability.

Preliminary data from the recent survey of functionally disabled
elderly in the community showed that 73 percent reported arthritis and
25 percent reported "numbness and stiffness" unrelated to arthritis. The
next-highest prevalence rates were for symptoms not necessarily associated with functional disability—sleep disturbance (42 percent) and con-
stipation (34 percent). Among this same population, 55 percent reported
having experienced circulatory problems in the extremities during the

Table 4-6. Number of persons affected and morbidity rates of the fifteen most prevalent chronic conditions for the total population and those aged 65 and over, 1981.

Condition	Number affected		Rate per 1,000 Age group		
	Total population	Total aged 65 & over	Under 45	45-64	65 & over
Arthritis	27,238,293	11,547,889	47.7	246.5	264.7
Hypertensive disease	25,523,526	9,406,958	54.2	243.7	378.6
Hearing impairments	18,665,650	7,051,238	43.8	142.9	283.8
Heart conditions	17,186,106	6,883,416	37.9	122.7	277.0
Chronic sinusitis	31,036,480	4,562,037	158.4	177.5	183.6
Visual impairments	9,083,717	3,395,397	27.4	55.2	136.6
Orthopedic impairments	18,416,051	3,185,397	90.5	117.5	128.2
Arteriosclerosis	3,398,230	2,410,125	0.5	21.3	97.0
Diabetes	5,499,737	2,073,037	8.6	56.9	83.4
Varicose veins	6,129,874	2,067,311	19.0	50.1	83.2
Hemorrhoids	8,848,365	1,637,487	43.7	66.6	65.9
Frequent constipation	3,599,159	1,471,915	9.2	22.4	59.2
Disease of the urinary system	5,689,273	1,395,187	25.8	31.7	56.1
Hay fever	17,873,906	1,290,449	100.2	77.5	51.9
Corns and callosities	4,289,880	1,289,933	14.0	35.8	51.9
Hernia of abdominal cavity	3,697,855	1,220,156	8.9	33.1	49.1

Source: National Center for Health Statistics, unpublished data from the National Health Interview Survey, 1981.

Table 4-7. Prevalence rates of leading chronic conditions in noninstitutionalized persons aged 65 and over, by sex, 1979.

	Male prevalence
Condition	Percentage
1. Arthritis	35.5
2. Hearing Impairment	32.7
3. Hypertension	31.5
4. Heart Conditions	26.6
5. Chronic sinusitis	13.5
6. Arteriosclerosis	12.2
7. Visual Impairment	12.0
8. Orthopedic Impairment	7.7
9. Diabetes	7.4
10. Hernia	7.1
11. Emphysema	6.8
12. Prostate Disease	5.8

	Female prevalence
Condition	Percentage
1. Arthritis	50.4
2. Hypertension	43.4
3. Heart Conditions	28.1
4. Hearing Impairment	25.0
5. Chronic sinusitis	17.1
6. Varicose veins	12.6
7. Arteriosclerosis	12.5
8. Visual Impairment	11.8
9. Orthopedic impairment	10.9
10. Diabetes	8.4
11. Constipation	8.0
12. Hemorrhoids	7.6

Source: National Center for Health Statistics, unpublished data from the National Health Interview Survey, 1979

previous 12 months, 48 percent reported having hypertension, and 37 percent had experienced a heart attack or other heart problem.[18]

Psychiatric Morbidity

Until recently little was known of the prevalence of psychiatric disorders in the community, but it has now been shown that for most conditions the incidence declines with age. High prevalence estimates of depressive illness in the elderly have been made from some studies, and suicide rates for white males aged 75 to 84 are higher than for all other population groups.[23,3] On the other hand, a recent multisite community survey found that both lifetime prevalence and the incidence of depression in the elderly living in the community was lower than for other age groups.[20,21]

Among those aged 65 and over in the noninstitutionalized population, severe cognitive impairment was the most common psychiatric disorder for men, followed by phobia and alcohol abuse or dependence. For women in this age group the most common disorder was phobia, followed by severe cognitive impairment.[21]

Estimates from the 1982 National Long-Term Care Survey showed that while absence of cognitive impairment declined with age, there was a very low prevalence of severe loss of cognitive functioning even among the very old.[19] These low rates undoubtedly occurred because the mental status questionnaire was not administered to the 26 percent of the survey population, that would have included the most severely impaired, for whom there was a proxy respondent.

It has been estimated from other studies that 20 percent of the total population aged 65 and over suffer from mild cognitive disability, while approximately 4 percent have what may be regarded as a malignant form of senile dementia, increasing in severity and prevalence with age. It is predicted that 20 percent of those aged 80 and over and 30 percent of those aged 85 and over will develop senile dementia of the Alzheimer type (SDAT).[10,22,23]

The available evidence indicates that mental disorders, including loss of cognitive functioning, are presently a leading cause of institutionalization. While it is not necessarily the primary reason for admission, a high proportion of the nursing home population was characterized as suffering from senile dementia (see Table 4-8). The prevalence was higher among women than men and increased with age, to 43 percent of women and 40 percent of men aged 85 and over.

Table 4-8. Prevalence rates of senility per 1,000 nursing home residents, by age and sex, 1977.

Age group	Males	Females
Under 65	45.7	66.1
65-74	182.1	241.6
75-84	319.9	382.9
85 & over	395.7	428.5

Source: National Center for Health Statistics: Hing, E., Characteristics of nursing home residents, health status and care received. National Nursing Home Survey, 1977. Vital and Health Statistics, Series 13, No. 51. DHHS Pub. No. (PHS)81-1712, Public Health Service. Washington, D.C., U.S. Government Printing Office, 1981.

It has been suggested that the administration of psychotropic drugs to the elderly induces symptoms interpreted as dementia,[24] and this may well be a contributory factor in the high prevalence of cognitive impairment in the nursing home population. Apart from nursing home residents, however, it was estimated in 1976 that an additional 75,000 persons aged 85 and over lived in other long-term care facilities, mostly chronic care mental hospitals.[25]

Table 4-9 illustrates the potential effect of population change on the prevalence of mental disorders between 1980 and 2005. It is predicted that while the prevalence of all mental disorders will increase in line with population growth, the rates for senile dementia will increase by a much greater magnitude as the age structure of the elderly population changes. An increasing number and proportion of the very old means that SDAT will be a growing problem in terms of appropriate provision of care and of increasing costs for such care, either institutional or community based.

Health expenditure data show that diseases of the circulatory system, which include heart disease, hypertension, and stroke, were responsible for the highest per capita personal heath care expenditures for the elderly of both sexes in 1980. The highest percentage of these expenditures was for acute hospital services, followed by nursing home care. For elderly females, mental disorders were the second most expensive condition; for elderly males, mental disorders ranked fifth in terms of personal health care expenditures.[26]

Many circulatory disorders are associated with costly high-technology medical intervention, while mental disorders lead to a high rate of custodial care in institutions. Arthritic, mental, and other disorders, leading to functional disability among the noninstitutionalized population, probably represent a much higher cost to individuals, families, and society in terms of the provision of nonreimbursed medical and supportive care than is reflected in medical expenditure data.

Functional Disability

Functional disability may result from physical and/or mental impairment and may be short or long term. There is no predictable relationship between morbidity and functional disability. The level of disability suffered as a result of arthritis, stroke, or any other condition may range from minimal, without any need for assistance, to total dependence on other individuals.

Two classifications relating to functional ability have been developed. Activities of Daily Living (ADL) refers to normal, everyday functions such as walking, bathing, toileting, dressing, and eating. Instrumental Activities of Daily Living (IADL) include home management activities such as grocery shopping, preparing meals, laundry, housework, managing money, using the telephone, and taking medicine. The list could be

Table 4-9. Illustration of the effect of population changes in the U.S. between 1980 and 2005 on selected indices of mental disorders, assuming 1980 rates applied to the projected population, by race, for 2005.

| | Number | | | | Percentage change 1980-2005 | |
| | White | | Black & other | | | |
	1980	2005	1980	2005	White	Black & other
Population	191,581,000	225,186,000	30,578,000	42,416,000	17.5	38.7
Cases of serious mental disorders (excluding senile dementia)	1,915,000	2,251,860	305,780	424,160	17.5	38.7
Senile dementia cases on a given day						
Total aged 65 & over	1,901,154	2,735,873	182,857	314,896	43.9	72.2
65-69 years	129,369	129,637	15,383	20,754	0.2	34.9
70-74	311,505	375,700	30,999	48,447	14.8	56.3
75-79	443,360	647,061	37,512	69,778	45.9	86.0
80 & over	1,016,920	1,601,475	98,963	175,917	57.7	77.7

Source: Kramer M., Trends in institutionalization and prevalence of mental disorders in nursing homes, National Conference on Mental Illness in Nursing Homes, Washington, D.C., October 4, 1983.

Table 4-10.   Rates of need for assistance in the noninstitutionalized elderly
population, by type of need and by age, 1979.

	Age group			
Type of need	65 & over	65-74	75-84	85 & over
	Percentage			
Needs help in one or more ADL*	9.02	5.26	11.40	34.84
Needs help in one or more IADL**	10.48	5.73	14.20	39.90
Bed-ridden	1.82	1.13	2.56	5.12
Has bowel or bladder device	2.97	0.05	1.08	2.85
Needs help of another person in one or more of the above areas	12.07	6.99	16.03	43.65

*   ADL need describes those who require assistance in walking, going outside,
bathing, dressing, toileting, getting in or out of bed or chair, and eating.

** IADL need describes those who require assistance with managing money, making
telephone calls, grocery shopping, preparing meals or doing routine household chores.

Source: National Center for Health Statistics. Feller B.A.: Americans needing help
to function at home. Advance Data from Vital and Health Statistics, No. 92 DHHS
Publication No. (PHS)83-1250, Public Health Service, Hyattsville, Md. September
1983.

extended to include an infinite range of activities; because of this,
reported prevalence rates for IADL limitations are higher than those for
ADL in most populations.[15,19]

Two recent national surveys of the noninstitutionalized population
produced somewhat different estimates of functional disability in the
elderly populations. The differences may be explained by the fact that one
was a household survey,[15,16] while the other surveyed elderly Medicare
enrollees.[17,19] There were other differences in the survey design, the first
focusing on "need for assistance" and the second on functional ability;
slightly different ADL and IADL classifications were also used. Both,
however, demonstrated clearly that functional disability and dependency
increase markedly with age.

Table 4-10 summarizes the results of the 1979 survey: 9 percent of the
total population aged 65 and over "need help" with one or more ADL's
and 11 percent with IADL's. Of those aged 65 to 74, only 5 percent had
ADL and less than 6 percent had IADL limitations; the percentage

increased to 35 and 40 percent for those aged 85 and over. The survey showed similar rates of increase with age for those who were bedridden, for bowel and bladder problems, and for "needing help from another person" for any one of these impairments.

Results from the 1982 survey of the noninstitutionalized population showed that 19 percent of elderly persons living in the community suffered functional impairment with regard to ADL's or IADL's of at least a three-month duration, representing about 5 million persons from the 27 million enrolled in Medicare. This study also demonstrated, as did the 1979 survey, that while the prevalence of functional impairment increases with age, from 13 percent of those aged 65 to 69 to 35 percent of those aged 85 and over, the highest number of disabled persons is in the younger age groups (see Table 4-11). In the total elderly Medicare population, prevalence of functional disability is higher among women than men (21 percent compared with 17 percent) and among black and other races than among whites (29 percent compared with 19 percent).[17] Prevalence rates of functional impairment increase with age for both blacks and whites but, in each age interval, disability rates are higher for blacks and other races than for whites. The rates for white men and women are relatively closer, differing by only 4.5 percentage points at ages 80 to 84. Elderly black women show markedly higher prevalence rates of functional disability compared with black men at each age interval except the very oldest.

Nearly 90 percent of the functionally disabled elderly reported one or more IADL limitations. As shown in Table 4-12, the percentage reporting no IADL limitations decreases with age, from 17 percent of those aged 65 to 69 to only 4 percent of those aged 85 and over, and the percentage reporting limitations in a higher number of IADL's increases with age. The percentage without IADL limitations was slightly higher for men than women and for whites than blacks. Table 4-13 shows the age and activity-specific prevalence rates for IADL limitations. Seventy-four percent of those reporting limitations in IADL were unable to do "heavy work," 57 percent to do "shopping for groceries," 47 percent to "go places or walk distances," while only 9 percent were unable to "get around inside." Those aged 85 and over had the highest IADL disability rates; 40 percent or more were unable to manage money, prepare meals, or do laundry.

By comparison with the rates of IADL impairment, 30 percent of the functionally disabled elderly reported having no ADL limitations, the rate declining from 39 percent of those aged 65 to 69 to 22 percent of those aged 85 and over; the percentage reporting higher disability levels increased with age (see Table 4-14). Table 4-15 shows the activity-specific distribution of ADL limitation: the highest overall impairment was with regard to "bathing" (42 percent), closely followed by "getting around inside" (40 percent). The lowest rates of impairment were reported for

Table 4-11. Number and percentage distribution of the total Medicare population and of functionally impaired elderly, living in the community, by age, race and sex, 1982.

| Age, race & sex | Total Medicare enrollment at July 1, 1982 (thousands) | Percentage | Persons with functional impairment | | Percentage of Medicare population |
			Number (thousands)	Percentage	
Total	26539.9	100.0	5073.9	100.0	19.1
Age 65-69	8652.1	32.6	1108.5	21.8	12.8
70-74	7021.6	26.5	1108.2	21.8	15.8
75-79	5063.9	19.1	1066.0	21.0	21.1
80-84	3184.9	12.0	885.5	17.5	27.8
85 & over	2617.4	9.9	905.7	17.9	34.5
White men					
Total	9369.9	100.0	1583.1	100.0	16.9
Age 65-69	3407.1	36.4	400.1	25.3	11.7
70-74	2589.5	27.6	373.4	23.6	14.4
75-79	1724.5	18.4	342.5	21.8	19.9
80-84	970.8	10.4	237.1	15.0	24.4
85 & over	678.1	7.2	230.0	14.5	33.9
White women					
Total	14026.6	100.0	2784.8	100.0	19.9
Age 65-69	4173.1	29.8	528.0	19.0	12.7
70-74	3564.1	25.4	565.1	20.3	15.9
75-79	2764.7	19.7	592.4	21.3	21.4
80-84	1879.1	18.4	542.1	19.5	28.9
85 & over	1645.6	11.7	567.2	20.4	34.5
Black & other race men					
Total	985.7	100.0	239.4	100.0	24.3
Age 65-69	354.4	36.0	68.6	28.7	19.4
70-74	276.3	28.0	65.9	27.5	23.9
75-79	184.8	18.7	41.0	17.1	22.2
80-84	100.7	10.2	29.9	12.5	29.7
85 & over	69.5	7.1	34.3	14.3	49.4
Black & other race women					
Total	1386.2	100.0	456.7	100.0	33.0
Age 65-69	449.0	32.4	111.8	24.5	24.9
70-74	362.3	26.1	103.7	22.7	28.6
75-79	264.5	19.1	90.2	19.8	34.1
80-84	166.7	12.0	76.7	16.8	46.0
85 & over	143.7	10.4	74.3	16.3	51.7

Source: Macken C.L., 1982 Long-Term Care Survey: national estimates of functional impairments among the elderly living in the community. Office of Research and Demonstrations, Health Care Financing Administration, (working paper), 1984.

Table 4-12. Percentage distribution of the number of IADL limitations reported by functionally disabled elderly living in the community, by age, race and sex, 1982

Number of IADL limitations reported

Age	0	1	2	3	4	5	6	7	8	9	10	Total
	Percentage of persons reporting limitations											
Total	10.5	12.9	12.2	12.3	12.0	9.2	6.7	7.2	7.1	6.5	3.5	100.0
Age 65 - 69	16.9	18.5	14.1	11.3	8.9	7.7	5.0	4.9	6.0	4.1	2.6	100.0
70 - 74	13.5	15.6	13.6	13.2	11.8	8.1	6.3	6.0	5.5	3.8	2.6	100.0
75 - 79	9.5	13.3	13.5	12.6	12.7	9.1	6.8	7.1	5.9	5.9	3.6	100.0
80 - 84	6.6	10.5	12.1	13.4	13.0	9.6	6.8	8.4	8.2	7.1	4.2	100.0
85 & over	3.9	4.6	6.8	11.1	14.0	12.3	8.5	10.5	10.5	12.9	4.9	100.0
Sex												
Male	13.3	14.2	12.4	9.3	8.5	8.0	6.5	7.2	9.2	7.3	4.2	100.0
Female	8.9	12.2	12.1	14.0	13.9	9.9	6.7	7.3	5.9	6.1	3.1	100.0
Race												
White	10.8	13.1	12.1	12.6	12.5	9.1	6.6	6.8	6.9	6.3	3.3	100.0
Black & other	8.7	11.6	12.9	10.2	7.9	10.3	6.4	10.2	8.3	8.4	5.3	100.0

Source: Macken C.L., Descriptive profile of the functionally impaired aged living in the community: findings from the 1982 Long-Term Care Survey. Office of Research and Demonstrations, Health Care Financing Administration, draft report, 1985.

"eating" (6 percent). Twenty-one percent reported problems "getting to the toilet," 24 percent problems with "continence," and 26 percent "getting in and out of bed."

A widely used Index of Independence in Activities of Daily Living (Index of ADL) has been developed. It ranks six sociobiological functions—bathing, dressing, toileting, transfer from bed and chair, continence, and feeding—in an hierarchical order to make comparisons between individuals and to rank them over time.[27] Individuals may be graded as "independent" or "dependent" in each activity, with a higher dependency score showing a higher level of functional disability.

A comparison of the noninstitutionalized with the nursing home population (Tables 4-14 and 6-9) shows far higher dependency rates in the nursing home than the noninstitutionalized population. Only 7.4 percent of the nursing home population aged 65 and over were ranked as "independent" and 25 percent as "dependent" in all ADL's compared with 33 percent and 2 percent, respectively, in the noninstitutionalized population. Nevertheless, because of the large size of the noninstitutionalized

Table 4-13. Percentage distribution of functionally disabled elderly, living in the community, by type of IADL limitation and by age, race and sex, 1982.

	Heavy work	Light work	Laundry	Preparing meals	Activity — Shopping for groceries	Getting around outside	Going places/ Walking distances	Managing money	Taking medicine
					Percentage				
Age									
Total	73.9	22.9	40.7	30.1	57.3	8.9	46.5	25.7	23.6
Age 65 - 69	70.0	19.3	32.3	22.9	44.9	6.3	36.5	17.6	18.0
70 - 74	72.6	20.2	36.4	24.5	50.0	8.5	40.1	18.9	18.9
75 - 79	73.6	21.9	38.3	28.8	57.0	7.6	47.3	24.6	23.3
80 - 84	74.3	23.7	44.8	32.8	62.1	10.1	53.4	30.5	26.4
85 & over	80.3	31.3	55.2	44.7	77.1	13.2	59.0	40.6	33.9
Sex									
Male	71.7	29.3	43.8	36.0	50.7	6.8	36.8	26.7	28.4
Female	75.1	19.4	39.0	26.8	61.1	10.2	51.9	25.2	20.9
Race									
White	74.7	22.8	40.4	29.7	57.8	9.0	46.8	25.2	23.2
Black & other	76.6	26.6	47.6	36.4	60.3	10.1	49.0	32.6	29.2

Source: Macken C.L. Descriptive profile of the functionally impaired aged living in the community: findings from the 1982 Long-Term Care Survey. Office of Research and Demonstrations, Health Care Financing Administration, draft report, 1985.

Table 4-14. Percentage distribution of number of ADL limitations reported by functionally disabled elderly living in the community, and by age, race and sex, 1982.

Number of ADL limitations reported

Age	0	1	2	3	4	5	6	7	Total
			Percentage of persons reporting limitations						
Total	33.3	22.7	14.9	9.8	7.4	6.0	3.8	2.1	100
Age 65 - 69	39.2	22.6	13.5	8.2	7.0	5.1	2.5	1.8	100
70 - 74	37.6	23.4	13.5	7.9	6.3	6.4	3.7	1.2	100
75 - 79	34.3	23.1	13.5	10.3	7.1	5.7	4.2	1.8	100
80 - 84	30.4	22.5	16.8	9.9	7.3	6.1	4.5	2.5	100
85 & over	22.1	21.6	18.3	13.4	9.5	7.1	4.4	3.5	100
Sex									
Male	37.5	22.9	11.9	8.4	7.4	6.4	3.6	1.9	100
Female	30.9	22.6	16.7	10.6	7.4	5.8	3.9	2.2	100
Race									
White	33.0	23.3	14.7	10.2	7.1	6.1	3.8	1.9	100
Black & other	35.2	18.2	16.9	7.4	9.4	5.6	3.6	3.8	100

Source: Macken C.L. Descriptive profile of the functionally impaired aged living in the community: findings from the 1982 Long-Term Care Survey. Office of Research and Demonstrations, Health Care Financing Administration, draft report, 1985.

population relative to that of nursing home residents, there are more severely disabled individuals living in the community. It is therefore apparent that factors other than functional dependency, such as family support, differentiate the institutionalized from the noninstitutionalized population.

A modified Index of ADL was used in a study designed to develop a technique for forecasting "active life expectancy" in the noninstitutionalized elderly of one state.[28,29] The expected years of "active life expectancy" decreased from 10 years for those aged 65 to 70 years to 2.9 years for those 85 and over. As shown in Table 4-16, those with a 15-month history of sustained independence before the study showed a lower probability of entering a nursing home and a higher probability of sustaining independence than those with a history of functional dependence among all older age groups. The study also demonstrated that those aged 85 and over have little chance of regaining functional capacity once it is compromised compared with other older age groups.[28,29]

Table 4-15. Percentage distribution of functionally disabled elderly, living in the community, reporting ADL limitations, by type of activity and by age, race and sex, 1982.

	Bathing	Dressing	Getting to the toilet	Getting in and out of bed	Getting around inside	Continence	Eating
			Percentage reporting limitation				
Total	42.1	19.5	20.9	26.0	40.1	24.2	6.0
Age 65 - 69	33.6	19.2	15.8	23.8	32.4	23.5	5.9
70 - 74	37.6	17.7	18.4	23.8	35.5	23.8	4.3
75 - 79	41.5	20.1	19.7	25.5	39.0	24.4	5.3
80 - 84	47.6	19.2	22.6	26.4	44.0	23.8	6.1
85 & over	53.2	21.9	29.8	31.5	52.5	25.9	8.9
Sex							
Male	37.9	22.0	14.6	24.7	38.6	20.7	7.0
Female	44.4	18.1	22.7	26.7	40.9	26.2	5.5
Race							
White	43.0	19.0	20.9	26.2	39.5	23.6	5.8
Black & other	35.8	22.8	20.5	27.8	44.1	28.7	7.4

Source: Macken, C.L., Descriptive profile of the functionally impaired aged living in the community: findings from the 1982 Long-Term Care Survey. Office of Research and Demonstrations, Health Care Financing Administration, draft report,1985.

Summary

Throughout this century life expectancy has increased as mortality rates have declined for men and women, both black and white. The improvements, however, have been greater for women than men and for whites than blacks, although there are some interesting inconsistencies with regard to the latter. In recent years death-rate declines have been as great if not greater for the very aged as for other age groups, leading to a growth in the proportion of very elderly in the population. Because of the differences in cause-specific rates of change in subgroups of the population, it is predicted that further mortality rate declines can be expected.

The unresolved question posed by increased life expectancy at all ages, however, is whether mortality reductions are associated with lower incidence of disease, reductions in the severity of disease, or medical intervention to postpone the lethal outcome of disease processes. For some diseases there has been an increase in the age at death, even though the incidence has been constant or increasing. Presently, the cardiovascular

Table 4-16. Probability of change in functional status* between years 1.25 and 6, by initial functional state and age for elderly persons living in the community: Massachusetts, 1974 - 1980.

Outcomes** functional state and age	(n)	Sustained or regained independence	Acquired or sustained dependence	Entered nursing home	Died
In community with 15-month history of sustained independence at year 1.25					
65-74	(670)	0.772	0.031	0.024	0.173
75-84	(304)	0.589	0.072	0.066	0.273
85 & over	(38)	0.289	0.053	0.158	0.500
In community with 15-month history of some functional dependence at year 1.25					
65-74	(56)	0.357	0.179	0.054	0.411
75-84	(54)	0.093	0.185	0.093	0.630
85 & over	(27)	0.000	0.222	0.185	0.593

* Functional status assessed on the Katz 4-item ADL scale with assessments for bathing, dressing, transference, and eating.

** Chi-square test statistic indicates that the effect of age on outcome is statistically significant at $P=.001$, regardless of functional status at year 1.25.

Source: Branch L.G., Katz S., Kniepmann K., Papsidero J.: A prospective study of functional status among community elders. American Journal of Public Health 74: 3: 266-268, 1984.

disorders incur major expenditures for medical intervention, but increasing knowledge of risk factors indicate that they may be amenable to future prevention. Some chronic diseases are not life threatening but result in high rates of functional disability. Loss of cognitive functioning with advancing age, for which preventive measures have not been identified, is distressing and costly to the individual, and to the family and results in high rates of institutionalization.

Levels of chronic morbidity and their association with age-related rates of functional disability are important in predicting the future health status of the elderly and consequent demand and expenditures for acute and long-term care. Mortality decline for the very old is a recent phenomenon; until recently, the elderly were treated as a homogeneous group in national morbidity surveys, even though they span a thirty-five year age range.

National studies of the elderly to develop age-specific morbidity and disability profiles have recently been undertaken; they have demonstrated that very few elderly individuals are without symptoms of at least one chronic disease and that functional disability increases substantially with each successive age group. It has also been shown that levels of functional impairment for all older age groups are higher for women than men, for blacks than whites, and for the poor than the nonpoor. The probability of achieving improvement in functional status also declines with advancing age. Nevertheless, studies show that the majority of the elderly, even in the very oldest age groups, do not report functional disability.

There are, however, no time series data to compare the experience of the present elderly population with that of the past or to predict how present experience will be reflected in future generations of elderly persons. Cohort differentials in cause-specific mortality and morbidity risks are not known and could only be developed through prospective longitudinal studies.

In the meantime, it is known that individuals do demonstrate a range of disease states in terms of age of onset and rate of disease progression, and an increase in the demand for services cannot necessarily be anticipated simply from the increase in the numbers of the very old. Nevertheless, the high age-related prevalence of chronic morbidity and lack of knowledge regarding risk factors for some of the more disabling physical and psychiatric disorders would support those who predict a future increase in overall levels of morbidity and associated functional disability in line with the increase in the number of individuals of advanced old age.

REFERENCES

1. National Center for Health Statistics. L. Fingerhut: Changes in mortality among the elderly, United States, 1940–78. Vital and Health Statistics, Series 3, No. 22, DHHS Pub. No. (PHS)82-1406. Public Health Service, Washington, D.C. U.S. Government Printing Office, March 1982.
2. Rosenwaike I., Yaffe N., Sagi P.C. The recent decline in mortality of the extreme aged: an analysis of statistical data. American Journal of Public Health 70: 1074–1080, 1980.
3. National Center for Health Statistics: Advance report, final mortality statistics, 1982. Monthly Vital Statistics Report, Vol 33, No. 9, Supp. DHHS Pub. No. (PHS)85-1120. Public Health Service, Hyattsville, Md. December 20, 1984.
4. U.S. Bureau of the Census, Current Population Reports, Series P-23, No. 138, Demographic and socioeconomic aspects of aging in the United States. Washington, D.C. U.S. Government Printing Office, 1984.
5. Fries J. F. Aging, natural death and the compression of morbidity. New England Journal of Medicine 303: 130–135, 1980.
6. Manton K. G. Changing concepts of morbidity and mortality in the elderly population. Milbank Memorial Fund Quarterly 60: 2: 183–244, 1982.
7. Soldo B. J., Manton K. G. The graying of America: demographic challenges

for socioeconomic planning. Socio-Economic Planning Sciences, 19: 4: 227–247, 1985.

8. Schneider E. L., Brody J. A. Aging, natural death and the compression of morbidity: another view. New England Journal of Medicine 309: 854–856, 1983.

9. Gruenberg E. M. The failures of success. Milbank Memorial Fund Quarterly 55: 3–24, 1977.

10. Kramer M. The rising pandemic of mental disorders and associated chronic diseases and disabilities. In Epidemiological Research as Basis for the Organization of Extramural Psychiatry. Acta Psychiatrica Scandinavica Suppl. 285: 62: 382–397, 1980.

11. Verbrugge L. M. Longer life but worsening health? Trends in health and mortality in middle aged and older persons. Milbank Memorial Fund Quarterly 62: 3: 475–519, 1984.

12. Colvez A., Blanchet M. Disability trends in the United States population, 1966–76: analysis of reported causes. American Journal of Public Health 71: 464–471, 1981.

13. National Center for Health Statistics: Health, United States, 1984. DHHS Pub. No. (PHS)85-1232, Public Health Service, Washington, D.C. U.S. Government Printing Office, December, 1984.

14. National Center for Health Statistics: Hing E. Characteristics of nursing home residents, health status and care received. National Nursing Home Survey, 1977. Vital and Health Statistics: Series 13, No. 51. DHHS Pub. No. (PHS)81-1712, Public Health Service, Washington D.C. U.S. Government Printing Office, 1981.

15. National Center for Health Statistics: Feller B. A. Americans needing help to function at home. Advance Data on Vital and Health Statistics: No. 92. DHHS Pub. No. (PHS)83-1250. Public Health Service, Hyattsville, Md. September 1983.

16. National Center for Health Statistics: Feller, B. A. Need for care among the noninstitutionalized elderly. Health, United States, 1983. DHHS Pub. No. (PHS)84-1232. Public Health Service, Washington, D.C. U.S. Government Printing Office, December 1983.

17. Macken C. L. 1982 Long-Term Care Survey: national estimates of functional impairments among the elderly living in the community. Office of Research and Demonstrations, Health Care Financing Administration, (working paper), 1984.

18. Soldo B. Preliminary data from the 1982 National Long-Term Care Survey, (unpublished).

19. Macken C. L. Descriptive profile of the functionally impaired aged living in the community: findings from the 1982 Long-Term Care Survey. Office of Research and Demonstrations, Health Care Financing Administration, draft report, 1985.

20. Robins L. N., Helzer J. E., Weissman M. M. et al. Lifetime prevalence of specific psychiatric disorders in three sites. Archives of General Psychiatry 41: 949–958, 1984.

21. Myers J. K., Weissman M. M., Tischler G. L. et al. Six month prevalence of psychiatric disorders in three communities, 1980–1982. Archives of General Psychiatry: 41: 959–967, 1984.

22. Sluss T. K., Gruenberg E. M., Kramer M. The use of longitudinal studies in the investigation of risk factors for Senile Dementia-Alzheimer Type. In Mortimer J. A., Schuman L. M. (eds), The Epidemiology of Dementia, New York: Oxford University Press, 1981.
23. Gurland B. J., Cross P. S. Epidemiology of psychopathology in old age: some implications for clinical services. The Psychiatric Clinics of North America 5: 11–26, 1982.
24. Blazer D. Depressive illness in late life. Presented to the Committee on Aging of the Institute of Medicine, July 1983.
25. Soldo B. J., Manton K. G. Modeling health status changes among the oldest old. Presented at the The Annual Meeting of the American Association for the Advancement of Science, May 26, 1984.
26. National Center for Health Statistics. Hodgson T. A., Kopstein A. N. Health care expenditures for major diseases. Health, United States, 1983, DHHS Pub. No. (PHS)84-1232, Public Health Service, Washington, D.C. U.S. Government Printing Office, December, 1983.
27. Katz S., Akpom C. A. A measure of primary sociobiological functions. International Journal of Health Services, 6: 493–507, 1976.
28. Katz S., Branch L. G., Branson M. H., Papsidero J. A., Greer D. S. Active life expectancy. The New England Journal of Medicine 309: 1218–1224, 1983.
29. Branch L. A., Katz S., Kniepman K., Papsidero J. A. A prospective study of functional status among community elders. American Journal of Public Health 74:3:266–268, 1984.

5

Health Care Expenditures and Utilization

Before 1929, nearly 90 percent of national health expenditures were from private funds, with federal expenditures confined generally to activities such as the control of communicable disease by the U.S. Public Health Service and the provision of health care to the armed forces. There was also limited federal and state funding of programs to promote the health of mothers and children and provide health care for the indigent.

The depression era followed by World War II expanded the federal government's role in funding both national and personal health care. Federal relief programs for the destitute unemployed in the early 1930's paid for medical care as part of assistance benefits. The Social Security Act of 1935 then made available federal grants to the states to develop health care for the unemployed and provided means-tested benefits under the Old Age Assistance program, enabling the elderly to pay for medical care.[1]

Individuals experienced extreme financial distress during the depression resulting in a deteriorating financial situation for health care providers and a need for new payment mechanisms in the voluntary and private sectors. In the 1930's the health insurance industry began to develop: Blue Cross was organized by the hospital associations, and Blue Shield prepayment plans for physician services were promoted under medical society sponsorship.[1]

During World War II, the federal government assumed a greater role in the direct provision of health care for the 12 million service personnel and their dependents and for agricultural and other workers important to a wartime economy.

In the postwar period former servicemen became eligible for a wide range of health care and other benefits under the Veterans Administration Act of 1946. In 1946 the Hill Burton Act was passed to provide federal subsidies to approved nonprofit hospital corporations for building and upgrading hospitals. This program was later extended to nursing homes and other nonhospital health facilities. Federal funding of medical research increased greatly through expanding the National Institutes of

79

Health, and grants to states were made to develop programs related to maternal and child health, rehabilitation, and health care for the indigent.[1]

For most of the population, however, there was no federal subsidy for personal health care; there was debate at this time on the feasibility and desirability of developing a program of national health insurance, but strong opposition to this proposal was mounted and the emphasis was placed on encouraging "voluntary" health insurance. This was increasingly negotiated as a "fringe benefit" with employers: by 1950, 51 percent of the population had some form of health insurance coverage compared with only 9 percent in 1940. Less than half of the elderly had any form of health insurance, however, and coverage was generally inadequate for all population groups.[1]

Between 1950 and 1960 national health expenditures more than doubled as technological innovation increased costs, particularly for acute hospital care, with the increased costs falling disproportionately on those with the highest utilization of health care—the elderly.

Federal grants to states for medical vendor payments for public assistance recipients were increased in 1956, and the Kerr-Mills Act of 1960 provided additional federal matching grants to states for medical vendor payments under their Old Age Assistance programs together with a new matching program, Medical Assistance for the Aged. This made payments to health care providers on behalf of those aged 65 and over who were judged to be "medically indigent" by the individual states.

After three years, only 28 of the 50 states had the program in operation; by this time, over 9 percent of the population was aged 65 and over. The elderly were becoming an important political force, and their middle class was voicing strong resistance to being forced into any form of "indigency" in order to meet health care costs.[1]

In 1965 Medicare, or Title XVIII of the Social Security Act, was passed to provide federally subsidized health insurance for the elderly. At the same time, Medicaid, Title XIX of the Social Security Act, was also passed. This extended the Kerr-Mills program of federal grants to states for the "medically indigent" under age 65. These 1965 amendments therefore provided the elderly with substantial protection against economic loss due to medical costs, particularly for acute hospital care.[1]

Medicare

Medicare was introduced on January 1, 1966. Private health insurance carriers, mainly Blue Cross and Blue Shield, were adopted as fiscal intermediaries with an open-ended responsibility for administering the program.

Medicare has two parts, each with its own trust fund. Part A, the hospital insurance (HI) program, pays for inpatient hospital services, skilled nursing home care, and home health services. In 1983 the HI provision requiring prior hospitalization for reimbursement of home health services was eliminated, as was the restriction on the number of visits, and a hospice benefit was introduced. Part B, the supplementary medical insurance (SMI) program, provides voluntary subsidized insurance for physician care, outpatient hospital visits, home health care, and other services.

Unlike other federal health programs, Medicare is not financed solely by general revenues. In 1983 84 percent of the income for the HI program came from a payroll tax levied on employers and employees. The SMI program is financed by monthly premium payments from individual enrollees and by general revenues, the share of the former increasing from 50 percent in 1971 to 74 percent in 1983.[2]

In 1973 Medicare coverage was extended to permanently disabled workers and their dependents eligible for Social Security benefits and to persons with end-stage renal disease. These beneficiaries now represent 10 percent of the Medicare population.

Medicare is oriented toward protecting individuals from major costs associated with acute episodes of illness rather than providing coverage for preventive or long-term care services. Nursing home and home health care are covered only for "skilled nursing" and rehabilitation services. Medicare was introduced in accordance with the principles of most private health insurance policies with "cost-based" retrospective reimbursement for providers and with deductibles, copayments, and coinsurance for the beneficiaries. Efforts to curb Medicare expenditures, however, have resulted in recent changes in reimbursement policies. In 1982 limits were imposed on total inpatient costs per hospital admission, and beneficiaries became entitled to enroll in health maintenance organizations (HMO's) and other prepaid comprehensive health care plans. The changes with regard to HMO enrollment were not implemented until April 1985. Beginning in October 1983, further prepayment initiatives were implemented in the form of "prospective payment," or predetermined reimbursement for each hospital admission on the basis of diagnosis-related groups (DRG's). The system was gradually introduced for all hospitals over a one-year period.[2] In July 1984 physician fees were frozen for fifteen months.

Medicaid

Medicaid was formally introduced in January 1966 as a joint federal-state program to provide medical assistance to certain categories of low-income people, including the aged, blind, disabled, and families with dependent children. These groups are called "categorically needy." States may also elect to extend Medicaid coverage to the "medically needy," with income limits determined by the individual state and to those who "spend down" their income because of high medical bills.

States were free to participate or not as they chose but, between 1965 and 1970, all states joined the program with the exception of Alaska and Arizona.[3] Alaska joined in 1973; in 1981 Arizona established a prepaid capitation program of health care for the poor, run as a demonstration program with support from the Health Care Financing Administration.[4]

Medicaid provides federal grants matching state expenditures, based on a formula related to the per capita income of the state, ranging from 50 to 78 percent in 1984; 83 percent is the maximum payable by law.[2]

As a state program, Medicaid is subject to wide variation in coverage and service provisions, but federal law requires participating states to provide certain services, including inpatient and outpatient hospital care, laboratory and X-ray services, skilled nursing home and home health care, and other specified services such as family planning. States may include additional services such as prescription drugs, eyeglasses, and dental care. Amendments in 1967 widened federal grants to Medicaid programs for service in intermediate care facilities (ICF's) as a lower-cost alternative to skilled nursing home care.

In contrast to Medicare, a high proportion of Medicaid expenditures are for long-term care in nursing homes or psychiatric hospitals and for home health services; the range of service provision and eligibility are determined by the individual states. The "medically needy" category, which has been adopted by the majority of the states, enables nursing home residents and others to become eligible for Medicaid reimbursements when they have "spent down" their assets.

Recent concern with cost restraint led to cutbacks of 3 to 4.5 percent in federal Medicaid reimbursement under the 1981 Omnibus Budget Reconciliation Act for fiscal years 1982 through 1984. Partial exemptions were made for states with very high unemployment and those that had implemented hospital cost reviews and programs to recover costs of fraud and abuse.[2]

Medicare and Medicaid—Dual Eligibility

Although Medicare and Medicaid are distinct programs, it was estimated in 1980 that 3.6 million elderly individuals, or 14 percent of the Medicare population, were eligible for both.[5] Under the Medicare law, states may buy coverage in the SMI program for persons eligible for cash or medical assistance. Medicare then makes the primary payment for Medicare-covered services; Medicaid pays any coinsurance or deductibles. In 1982 all states except Louisiana, Oregon, and Wyoming had buy-in agreements for their Medicaid enrollees.

DATA SOURCES

Sources of information for the tables presented in this chapter are as follows.

National health expenditure and utilization data are collected, analyzed, and disseminated by the Bureau of Data Management and Strategy and the Division of Medical Cost Estimates, both divisions of the Office of Financial and Actuarial Analysis of the Health Care Financing Administration.

Data are also available from the National Health Care Expenditures Study 1977–1978, carried out by the National Center for Health Services Research,[6] and the National Medical Care Utilization and Expenditure Survey, carried out by the National Center for Health Statistics in 1980.[7] The former was a survey of 14,000 randomly selected households, interviewed six times during an eighteen-month period; the latter was also a national, longitudinal household survey of the noninstitutionalized population, together with a survey of Medicaid-eligible households in four states.

National Health Expenditures

National health expenditures include those for personal health care together with the costs of public health services, administration, construction of medical facilities, and research. (The latter excludès research funded by drug companies and manufacturers of medical equipment, since total costs are included in the final product price.)

As a proportion of gross national product (GNP), national health expenditures increased from 3.5 percent in 1929 to 6 percent in 1965, and from 6.4 percent in 1967 to 10.8 percent in 1983 (see Table 5-1). GNP grew at an average rate of 9.4 percent per year between 1970 and 1983; health expenditure growth averaged 12.8 percent per year, with a 400-percent increase in per capita expenditures during this time.

Table 5-1 also demonstrates the change in the distribution of funding of health care between the private and public sectors. Private expenditures fell from over 86 percent of the total in 1929 to 73 percent in 1950, rose again to over 75 percent in 1960, and showed a major decline with the introduction of Medicare and Medicaid between 1965 and 1967. This trend continued down, to 57 percent between 1967 and 1980, but showed a slight rise to 58 percent in 1983.

Federal funding of total national health expenditures increased (by 43 percent) from 13 to 23 percent between 1965, the year before the Medicare and Medicaid programs were implemented, and 1967, the year after. It has risen constantly to reach 29 percent of total health expenditures in 1983. By contrast, state expenditures have varied little as a percentage of national health expenditures, fluctuating in the range of 13 to 14.5 percent between 1950 and 1983, although the one percentage point drop between 1980 and 1983, from 14 to 13 percent, is reflected in the increase in private expenditures.

Per capita private expenditures for health care rose 560 percent between 1967 and 1983. Per capita public expenditures rose 650 percent during the same period.

Table 5-1. Aggregate and per capita national health expenditures by source of funds and as a percentage of gross national product, selected years 1929-1983.

	1983	1980	1978	1975	1973	1970
National Health Expenditures (billions of dollars)	$355.4	$248.0	$190.0	$132.7	$103.4	$74.7
As a percentage of the GNP	10.8	9.4	8.8	8.6	7.8	7.5
Sources of funds:						
Private expenditures	$206.6	$142.2	$110.1	$76.3	$64.0	$46.9
Public expenditures	148.8	105.8	79.9	56.4	39.4	27.8
Federal expenditures	102.7	71.1	53.8	37.1	25.2	17.7
State/local expenditures	46.1	34.8	26.1	19.3	14.2	10.1
Per capita expenditures *	$1,459	$1,049	$822	$590	$468	$358
Private expenditures	848	601	476	340	290	225
Public expenditures	611	448	346	251	178	133
Percentage distribution of funds	100.0	100.0	100.0	100.0	100.0	100.0
Private funds	58.1	57.3	57.9	57.5	61.9	62.8
Public funds	41.9	42.7	42.1	42.5	38.1	37.2
Federal funds	28.9	28.7	28.4	28.0	24.4	23.6
State/local funds	13.0	14.0	13.7	14.5	13.7	13.6
Addenda:						
Gross National Product (billions of dollars)	3304.8	2631.7	2163.9	1549.2	1326.4	992.7
Population (millions)	243.6	236.4	231.3	224.8	220.8	208.6

	1967	1965	1960	1950	1940	1929
National Health Expenditures (billions of dollars)	$51.3	$41.7	$26.9	$12.7	$4.0	$3.6
As a percentage of the GNP	6.4	6.0	5.3	4.4	4.0	3.5
Sources of funds:						
Private expenditures	32.3	31.0	20.3	9.2	3.2	3.2
Public expenditures	19.0	10.8	6.6	3.4	0.8	0.5
Federal expenditures	11.9	5.5	3.0	1.6	NA	NA
State/local expenditures	7.1	5.3	3.6	1.8	NA	NA
Per capita expenditures *	254	211	146	82	30	29
Private expenditures	160	156	110	60	24	25
Public expenditures	94	55	36	22	6	4
Percentage distribution of funds	100.0	100.0	100.0	100.0	100.0	100.0
Private funds	63.0	74.1	75.3	72.8	79.7	86.4
Public funds	37.0	25.9	24.7	27.2	20.3	13.6
Federal funds	23.3	13.3	11.2	12.8	NA	NA
State/local funds	13.7	12.6	13.5	14.4	NA	NA
Addenda:						
Gross National Product (billions)	799.6	691.0	506.5	286.5	100.0	103.4
Population (millions)	202.3	197.9	183.8	154.7	134.6	123.7

* Based on July 1 Social Security area population estimates.

NA: Data not available.

Source: Office of Financial and Actuarial Analysis, Bureau of Data Management and Strategy, Health Care Financing Administration, 1984.

Table 5-2. Percentage distribution of personal health care expenditures by source of funds, selected years 1929-1983.

| | | | All third parties | | | | | |
| | | | Private | | | Public | | |
Year	Total	Patient direct payments	Total	Health insurance	Other	Total	Federal	State & local
1929	100.0	88.4	11.6	*	2.6	9.0	2.7	6.3
1935	100.0	82.4	17.6	*	2.8	14.7	3.4	11.3
1940	100.0	81.3	18.7	*	2.6	16.1	4.1	12.0
1950	100.0	65.5	34.5	9.1	2.9	22.4	10.4	12.0
1955	100.0	58.1	41.9	16.1	2.8	23.0	10.5	12.5
1960	100.0	54.9	45.1	21.1	2.3	21.8	9.3	12.5
1965	100.0	51.6	48.4	24.2	2.2	22.0	10.1	11.9
1966	100.0	49.5	50.5	22.9	2.1	25.5	13.2	12.3
1967	100.0	42.6	57.4	21.6	1.9	33.9	21.3	12.6
1968	100.0	41.2	58.8	21.7	1.8	35.3	22.6	12.7
1969	100.0	40.4	59.6	22.7	1.6	35.3	23.1	12.3
1970	100.0	40.5	59.5	23.4	1.7	34.3	22.2	12.1
1971	100.0	38.9	61.1	23.8	1.8	35.5	23.2	12.3
1972	100.0	38.0	62.0	23.6	2.5	35.8	23.5	12.3
1973	100.0	37.4	62.6	24.0	2.5	36.1	23.7	12.4
1974	100.0	35.3	64.7	24.8	1.5	38.4	25.9	12.6
1975	100.0	32.5	67.5	26.7	1.3	39.5	26.8	12.7
1976	100.0	31.6	68.4	28.3	1.2	38.7	27.2	11.5
1977	100.0	31.1	68.9	28.8	1.3	38.8	27.5	11.3
1978	100.0	30.3	69.7	29.3	1.2	39.2	27.7	11.5
1979	100.0	29.4	70.6	30.0	1.2	39.3	28.1	11.2
1980	100.0	28.5	71.5	30.7	1.2	39.6	28.5	11.0
1981	100.0	27.9	72.1	31.1	1.2	39.8	29.3	10.4
1982	100.0	27.1	72.9	31.9	1.2	39.8	29.5	10.3
1983	100.0	27.2	72.8	31.9	1.2	39.7	29.7	10.1

* Included with direct payments; separate data not available.

Source: Office of Financial and Actuarial Analysis, Bureau of Data Management and Strategy, Health Care Financing Review 6: 2: 1-29, 1984.

The rate of growth in health expenditures is expected to moderate through the 1980's due to lower inflation, but factors likely to stimulate growth include the continued aging of the population, technological innovation, and increasing health manpower. Total health expenditures are projected to rise from $355 billion in 1983 to $756 billion in 1990, representing 12 percent of GNP.[8]

Personal Health Care Expenditures

Table 5-2 shows changes in the distribution of personal health care expenditures between 1929 and 1983. There was a steady decline during this period in the proportion of direct payments for personal health care; this was in inverse relationship to the increase in third-party payments from 12 to 73 percent.

The growth of the private health insurance sector is demonstrated by the constant increase in the share of private health insurance reimbursements from 1950 to 1983, except for a slight decline from 24 to 22 percent between 1965 and 1967 when Medicare came into effect. By 1983 private insurance accounted for 32 percent of expenditures.

Federal payments for personal health care declined somewhat in the 1950's; they increased from 10 percent in 1965, the year before Medicare and Medicaid were introduced, to 30 percent in 1983. The introduction of Medicare and Medicaid had little impact on state expenditures, which declined from 13 percent in 1975 to 10 percent in 1983.

State Variations

Some insight into the factors that influence health care expenditures may be gained by examining state variations in expenditures and resources.

It has been theorized that physicians are the most influential group in determining the size and shape of the health care sector.[2,9] A study of personal health care data for 1978 demonstrated that the states with the highest per capita expenditures for health care—Massachusetts, California, Connecticut, and New York—also had the highest ratio of physicians to population.[9]

On the other hand, the states with the highest per capita expenditures were not the ones that experienced the highest rate of growth in the period from the introduction of Medicare and Medicaid in 1966 to 1978. Growth was greatest in the Southeast, where per capita expenditures quadrupled: Mississippi led the nation with an average annual growth rate of 14 percent, followed by Alabama with 13 percent.[11] The introduction of Medicare as a "universal" benefit for the elderly, with the shift from private to public funding, undoubtedly increased access to more expensive medical care, and the impact naturally would have been greatest for the population in states with the lowest per capita incomes.

Changes in population size and the "aging" of the population may also affect the growth of expenditures for health care.[8] As shown in Table 5-3, the average annual growth of total personal health care expenditures was 12.8 percent, of which 1.1 percent can be attributed to population increases and 0.6 percent to the "aging" of the population. Although these factors account for a small percentage of the growth rate, they do explain a high proportion of the variation between states.

Slower population growth in many of the northern, eastern, and midwestern states was also associated with a slower rate of growth in health care expenditures between 1966 and 1978. By contrast, Arizona, Nevada, and Florida ranked highest in the nation in the growth of personal health

Table 5-3. Average annual growth in personal health expenditures, total population growth, growth of population aged 65 and over, and effect of aging on health expenditures, by state, 1966-1978

| State | Average annual percentage growth 1966-1978 | | | Effect of aging on health expenditures 1966-1978 |
	Personal health expenditures	Total population	Aged 65 & over	
United States	12.8	1.1	2.2	0.6
Alabama	14.0	0.8	2.8	0.8
Alaska	14.0	3.3	5.9	0.7
Arizona	15.6	3.8	6.7	1.0
Arkansas	14.2	1.4	2.5	0.7
California	13.4	1.6	2.8	0.6
Colorado	12.8	2.7	2.4	0.4
Connecticut	11.6	0.5	2.2	0.7
Delaware	12.2	1.2	2.7	0.7
District of Columbia	10.5	-1.2	0.4	0.7
Florida	16.3	3.4	6.2	1.1
Georgia	14.6	1.6	3.1	0.7
Hawaii	13.6	2.3	5.3	0.9
Idaho	14.0	2.4	2.7	0.5
Illinois	11.8	0.4	1.2	0.5
Indiana	12.4	0.7	1.5	0.5
Iowa	12.0	0.5	0.8	0.0
Kansas	12.8	0.5	1.3	0.6
Kentucky	12.3	1.2	1.6	0.5
Louisiana	13.8	1.2	2.5	0.7
Maine	13.0	0.9	1.3	0.4
Maryland	13.3	1.1	3.0	0.7
Massachusetts	11.8	0.3	1.2	0.5
Michigan	12.4	0.7	1.7	0.6
Minnesota	11.7	0.9	1.4	0.5
Mississippi	15.0	0.9	2.2	0.7
Missouri	12.9	0.6	1.4	0.5
Montana	12.5	0.9	1.7	0.6
Nebraska	12.4	0.6	1.2	0.5
Nevada	17.3	4.1	7.3	0.9
New Hampshire	12.7	2.3	2.0	0.3
New Jersey	12.0	0.6	2.1	0.6
New Mexico	13.4	1.8	4.4	1.0
New York	10.6	-0.1	0.9	0.5
North Carolina	13.7	1.3	3.4	0.8
North Dakota	12.5	0.1	1.8	0.8
Ohio	12.2	0.4	1.4	0.6
Oklahoma	12.9	1.4	2.2	0.5
Oregon	13.8	2.0	2.8	0.5
Pennsylvania	11.9	0.1	1.6	0.6
Rhode Island	11.8	0.5	1.9	0.6
South Carolina	14.6	1.6	3.4	0.8
South Dakota	11.7	0.1	1.1	0.6
Tennessee	13.9	1.3	2.6	0.6
Texas	14.2	2.1	3.1	0.6
Utah	13.7	2.5	3.3	0.5
Vermont	12.1	1.6	1.3	0.3
Virginia	14.3	1.4	3.0	0.7
Washington	12.6	2.0	2.5	0.5
West Virginia	12.5	0.7	1.4	0.6
Wisconsin	12.5	0.7	1.7	0.6
Wyoming	11.6	2.4	1.8	0.4

Source: Levit K.R. Personal Health Care Expenditures by State, Selected Years, 1966-1978. Health Care Financing Review 4: 2: 1-45, 1982.

care spending and in annual population growth and growth of the population aged 65 and over.

Age Group Differences

During recent years health care expenditures for the elderly have been growing at a higher rate than for other sectors of the population. In 1978 per capita spending on health care for the elderly was seven times as great as for persons under 19 and two and a half times as great as for those aged 19 to 64. These differences are now estimated to have increased.[3,10]

Total health care expenditures for those aged 65 and over doubled between 1965 and 1970, from $8.8 billion to $17.3 billion; they increased another 700 percent between 1970 and 1984, to $119.9 billion (see Table 5.4).[3,10] Besides the major change in the funding of health care for the elderly from the private to the public sector, there was a shift in the distribution of resources toward institutional care: the hospital and nursing home sectors accounted for 66 percent of expenditures in 1984 compared with 58 percent in 1965.

Hospitalization rates have increased for all age groups since 1965, but there was a 35-percent increase in the hospitalization rate for individuals aged 65 and over between 1967 and 1979 compared with an 11-percent increase for the rest of the population. At the same time, there was a 58-percent increase in the rate of surgical operations for those aged 65 and over compared with a 24-percent increase for the rest of the population.[11]

While the elderly have a higher rate of hospital admission, longer lengths of stay, and greater use of physician services compared with other population groups,[3,11] there are major differences in utilization and expenditures within the elderly population. In 1976 those aged 85 and over used 5,484 days of hospital care per 1,000 persons compared with 3,684 for the elderly population as a whole, and the very aged have been shown to have higher costs associated with surviving an acute episode of illness than the less aged.[3,12]

Of public health expenditures for the elderly in 1984, Medicare will be responsible for 73 percent, Medicaid 19 percent, and the VA and other public programs 8 percent.[11] Of the total per capita expenditures on behalf of the elderly, Medicare will fund nearly 50 percent and Medicaid another 13 percent (see Table 5-5).

Medicare: Utilization and Expenditures

Total Medicare expenditures grew by 1,300 percent between 1967 and 1983: hospital reimbursements accounted for 70 percent or more of this spending in each time period, but declined from a high of nearly 75 percent in 1975 to 70 percent in 1983 (see Table 5-6). There has been a constant decrease in the proportion of Medicare expenditures for nursing

Table 5-4. Aggregate health care expenditures and percentage distribution for the population aged 65 and over, by type of expenditure and source of funds, selected years 1965 to 1984.

(Numbers in millions)

	Total expenditures	Private expenditures	Percent of total	Public expenditures	Percentage of total
1965 Total	$8,869	$6,213	70.1	$2,656	29.9
Hospital	3,296	1,677	50.9	1,619	49.1
Physician	1,737	1,617	93.1	120	6.9
Nursing home	1,825	1,187	65.0	638	35.0
Other	2,011	1,732	86.1	279	13.9
1970 Total	17,270	6,694	38.8	10,577	61.2
Hospital	7,054	806	11.4	6,248	88.6
Physician	3,030	1,166	38.5	1,864	61.5
Nursing home	4,144	2,255	54.4	1,889	45.6
Other	3,042	2,467	81.1	576	18.9
1976 Total	37,674	13,372	35.5	24,302	64.5
Hospital	16,305	1,831	11.2	14,474	88.8
Physician	6,505	2,746	42.2	3,759	57.8
Nursing home	9,395	4,693	50.0	4,702	50.0
Other	5,469	4,102	75.0	1,367	25.0

1977 Total	43,425	15,669	36.1	27,756	63.9
Hospital	18,906	2,319	12.3	16,587	87.7
Physician	7,782	3,323	42.7	4,458	57.3
Nursing home	10,696	5,424	50.7	5,272	49.3
Other	6,041	4,603	76.2	1,438	23.8
1981 Total	83,200	30,000	36.0	53,200	64.0
Hospital	36,600	5,300	14.5	31,300	85.5
Physician	15,600	6,600	42.3	9,000	57.7
Nursing home	19,400	9,600	49.5	9,800	50.5
Other	11,600	8,500	73.3	3,100	26.7
1984 Total	119,872	39,341	32.8	80,531	67.2
Hospital	54,200	6,160	11.4	48,040	88.6
Physician	24,770	9,827	39.7	14,943	60.3
Nursing home	25,105	13,083	51.9	12,067	48.1
Other	15,798	10,316	65.3	5,482	34.7

Source: Fisher C., Differences by age groups in health care spending. Health Care Financing Review 1: 4: 65-90, 1980, and Waldo D.R. and Lazenby H.C., Demographic characteristics and health care use and expenditures by the aged in the United States: 1977 - 1984. Health Care Financing Review 6: 1: 1-29, 1984. 1981 data from the Bureau of Data Management and Strategy, Health Care Financing Administration (unpublished data).

Table 5-5. Total per capita personal health care expenditures and percentage distribution for individuals aged 65 and over, by source of funds and type of service, 1984.

Type of service

Source of funds	Total per capita	Total care	Hospital	Physician	Nursing home	Other care
Total per capita	$4,202	100.0	45.2	20.7	20.9	13.2
Private	1,379	100.0	15.7	25.0	33.1	26.2
Consumer	1,363	100.0	15.3	25.3	33.1	26.3
Out-of-pocket	1,059	100.0	5.6	21.4	41.6	31.3
Insurance	304	100.0	49.2	38.6	3.3	8.9
Other private	16	100.0	42.1	1.9	39.1	17.0
Government	2,823	100.0	59.7	18.6	15.0	6.8
Medicare	2,051	100.0	69.2	24.5	0.9	5.4
Medicaid	536	100.0	17.0	3.1	68.1	11.8
Other government	236	100.0	73.2	2.4	16.5	7.9

Source of funds	Total care	Hospital	Physician	Nursing home	Other care
Total per capita	100.0	100.0	100.0	100.0	100.0
Private	32.8	11.4	39.7	51.9	65.3
Consumer	32.4	11.0	39.6	51.2	64.8
Out-of-pocket	25.2	3.1	26.1	50.1	59.9
Insurance	7.2	7.9	13.5	1.1	4.9
Other private	0.4	0.4	0.0	0.7	0.5
Government	67.2	88.6	60.3	48.1	34.7
Medicare	48.8	74.8	57.8	2.1	19.9
Medicaid	12.8	4.8	1.9	41.5	11.4
Other government	5.6	9.1	0.7	4.4	3.4

Source: Office of Financial and Actuarial Analysis, Bureau of Data Management and Strategy, Health Care Financing Administration, 1985.

Table 5-6. Medicare expenditures and percentage distribution by type of service, selected years 1967-1983.

Type of service	Year						
	1967	1970	1975	1979	1980	1981	1983
	Amount in billions						
Total	$4.5	$7.1	$15.6	$29.3	$35.7	$43.5	$57.4
	Percentage						
All services	100.0	100.0	100.0	100.0	100.0	100.0	100.0
Hospital care	69.0	71.8	74.8	72.1	72.6	72.0	70.3
Physician services	24.7	22.5	21.3	22.1	21.8	22.3	23.3
Nursing home care	4.6	4.2	1.9	1.4	1.1	0.9	0.9
Other services *	1.7	1.4	1.9	4.4	4.5	4.6	5.5

* Other services include home health agencies, home health services,

Source: National Center for Health Statistics, Health, United States 1984. DHHS Pub. No. (PHS)84-1232, Public Health Service. Washington, D.C., U.S. Government Printing Office, December 1984.

home care, from 4.6 percent of the total budget in 1967 to less than 1 percent in 1983.

In 1967, the first full year after Medicare was introduced, there were 19.5 million enrollees. As shown in Table 5-7, there has been an average annual increase of 2 percent, to 27.1 million enrollees in 1983. Utilization, however, increased at a higher rate than enrollment, so that there was a 5.9 percent annual increase in the number of persons served between 1967 and 1982. There was a 2.5 percent average annual decline in the use of skilled nursing facilities between 1967 and 1982, but the apparent decline in the utilization of SMI home health agency services was brought about by changes in the benefit and the switching of reimbursement from SMI to HI.

The average annual Medicare reimbursement for aged beneficiaries grew by 16.4 percent between 1967 and 1982 and by 20.4 percent between 1981 and 1982 (see Table 5-8). The highest rate of increase was for hospital outpatient and HI home health agency services.

(In addition to aged enrollees, the number of disabled enrollees increased at an average rate of 5.5 percent between 1974 and 1982, to nearly 3 million; annual reimbursements grew at an average annual rate of 24.8 percent during this period, and by 16.1 percent between 1981 and 1982.)

Table 5-7. Medicare utilization: number of aged beneficiaries enrolled and served and percentage change by type of service, 1967, 1980, 1981 and 1982.

Type of beneficiary & type of service	1967	1980	1981	1982	1967-82	1981-82
					Annual percentage change	
Persons enrolled	Number in thousands					
Hospital Insurance (HI) and/or Supplementary Medical Insurance (SMI)	19,521	25,515	26,011	26,540	2.1	2.0
Hospital Insurance	19,494	25,104	25,591	26,115	2.0	2.0
Supplementary Medical Insurance	17,893	24,680	25,182	25,707	2.4	2.1
Persons served						
All covered services	7,154	16,271	17,036	17,023	5.9	-0.1
Hospital insurance *	3,960	6,024	6,229	6,548	3.4	5.1
Inpatient hospital	3,601	5,951	6,072	6,338	3.8	4.4
Skilled nursing facility	354	248	243	244	-2.5	0.4
Home health agency	126	675	881	1,074	15.4	21.9
Supplementary medical insurance*	6,523	16,099	16,858	16,807	6.5	-0.3
Physician and other medical	6,415	15,627	16,380	16,346	6.4	-0.2
Outpatient hospital *	1,511	6,629	7,096	7,465	11.2	5.2
Home health agency	118	302	187	17	-12.1	-90.9
Persons served per 1000 enrolled						
All covered services	366.5	637.7	655.0	641.4	3.8	-2.1
Hospital insurance *	203.1	240.0	243.4	250.7	1.4	3.0
Inpatient hospital	184.7	237.1	237.3	242.7	1.8	2.3
Skilled nursing facility	18.2	9.9	9.5	9.3	-4.4	-2.1
Home health agency	6.5	26.9	34.4	41.1	13.1	19.5
Supplementary medical insurance*	364.5	652.3	669.5	653.8	4.0	-2.3
Physician and other medical	358.5	633.2	650.5	635.9	3.9	-2.2
Outpatient hospital *	77.4	268.6	281.8	290.4	9.2	3.1
Home health agency	6.6	12.2	7.4	0.7	-13.9	-90.5

* Prior to April 1, 1968 outpatient hospital services were covered by HI and SMI. All outpatient hospital services for 1967 are shown as SMI services for purposes of comparison. HI and SMI totals, however, include services paid under their respective trust funds.

Source: Office of Statistics and Data Management, Bureau of Data Management and Strategy, Health Care Financing Administration, 1984.

Table 5-8. Medicare utilization: amount reimbursed for aged beneficiaries and percentage change by type of service, 1967, 1980, 1981 and 1982.

Reimbursement	1967	1980	1981	1982	1967-1982	1981-1982
					Annual percent change	
	Amount in millions **					
All covered services	$4,239	$29,134	$34,490	$41,526	16.4	20.4
Hospital Insurance (HI)*	2,967	20,353	24,153	29,214	16.5	21.0
Inpatient hospital	2,659	19,583	23,111	27,834	16.9	20.4
Skilled nursing facility	274	331	361	388	2.3	7.5
Home health agency	26	440	682	992	27.5	45.5
Supplementary Medical Insurance (SMI)*	1,272	8,781	10,336	12,311	16.3	19.1
Physician and other medical	1,224	7,361	8,688	10,311	15.3	18.7
Outpatient hospital *	38	1,261	1,557	1,982	30.2	27.3
Home health agency	17	159	91	19	0.7	-79.1
Reimbursement per person served						
All covered services	$592	$1,791	$2,024	$2,439	9.9	20.5
Hospital Insurance (HI)*	749	3,379	3,877	4,462	12.6	15.1
Inpatient hospital	738	3,291	3,806	4,391	12.6	15.4
Skilled nursing facility	774	1,336	1,486	1,591	4.9	7.1
Home health agency	204	652	774	923	10.6	19.3
Supplementary Medical Insurance (SMI)*	195	545	613	733	9.2	19.6
Physician and other medical	191	471	530	631	8.3	19.1
Outpatient hospital *	25	190	219	265	17.0	21.0
Home health agency	145	526	488	1,091	14.4	123.6

* Prior to April 1, 1968 outpatient hospital services were covered by HI and SMI. All outpatient hospital services for 1967 are shown as SMI services for purposes of comparison. HI and SMI totals, however, include services paid under their respective trust funds.

** Parts may not add to total due to rounding.

Source: Office of Statistics and Data Management, Bureau of Data Management and Strategy, Health Care Financing Administration, 1984.

95

Table 5-9. Selected measures of use of Medicare benefits by decedents in their last year of life, and by survivors, according to age, 1978.

Survival status

Age	Decedents	Survivors	Decedents to survivors ratio
	Persons served* as a percentage of enrollees		
67 & over	92	58	1.6
67-69	91	53	1.7
70-74	93	56	1.6
75-79	93	60	1.5
80-84	93	62	1.5
85 & over	91	63	1.5
	Reimbursement per person served		
67 & over	$4,909	$1,253	3.9
67-69	6,354	1,109	5.7
70-74	5,897	1,181	5.0
75-79	5,433	1,285	4.2
80-84	4,617	1,391	3.3
85 & over	3,598	1,421	2.5
	Reimbursement per enrollee		
67 & over	$4,527	$729	6.2
67-69	5,801	592	9.8
70-74	5,466	668	8.2
75-79	5,056	771	6.5
80-84	4,274	859	5.0
85 & over	3,285	889	3.7

* Persons served are enrollees with some Medicare reimbursement.

NOTE: Data are derived from the Medicare Statistical System and are expressed in 1978 dollars.

Source: National Center for Health Statistics, Lubitz J., Prihoda R., Use and costs of Medicare services in the last years of life. Health, United States 1983. DHHS Pub. No. (PHS)84-1232, Public Health Service. Washington, D.C., U.S. Government Printing Office, December 1983.

Medicare reimbursements for the 5.2 percent of aged enrollees who died in 1978 represented 28.2 percent of program expenditures on behalf of the elderly.[12] Table 5-9 demonstrates that reimbursements in the last year of life for those who died were 6.2 times greater than for those who survived. Of those who survived, the reimbursements for those aged 85 and over were 28 percent greater than for those aged 67 to 69 years.[12] Table 5-10 illustrates the low Medicare reimbursements per enrollee for nursing home and home health care compared with the 77 percent of reimbursements for hospital care for those who died.

Table 5-10. Medicare reimbursement per enrollee and percentage distribution of total reimbursement for decedents in the last and second-to-last years of life, and for survivors, by type of service, in 1977 and 1978.

Year and type of service	Survival status				Ratio of reimbursement per enrollee of decedents to survivors
	Decedents		Survivors		
	Amount	Percentage distribution	Amount	Percentage distribution	
Last year (1978)					
All services	$4,527	100	$729	100	6.2
Hospital	3,484	77	478	66	7.3
Physician and other medical	769	17	198	27	3.9
Skilled nursing facility	89	2	7	1	12.7
Hospital outpatient	101	2	30	4	3.4
Home health agency	83	2	16	2	5.2
Second-to-last year (1977)					
All services	$1,481	100	$635	100	2.3
Hospital	1,008	68	416	65	2.4
Physician and other medical	338	23	176	28	1.9
Skilled nursing facility	33	2	8	1	4.1
Hospital outpatient	59	4	24	4	2.5
Home health agency	43	3	12	2	3.6

Notes: Data are derived from the Medicare Statistical System and are expressed in 1978 dollars. Details may not add to total because of rounding.

Source: National Center for Health Statistics, Lubitz J., Prihoda R., Use and costs of Medicare services in the last years of life. Health, United States 1983. DHHS Pub. No. (PHS)84-1232, Public Health Service. Washington, D.C., U.S. Government Printing Office, December 1983.

An analysis of 1976 Medicare data relating to the costs of hospital, nursing home, and home health agency care showed that episodes of illness that required only hospital care were substantially cheaper than those associated with posthospital care, and that utilization of posthospital services increased with age: 16 percent of those aged 85 and over used posthospital services compared with only 5 percent of those aged 65 to 69.[13] This, however, does not answer questions raised about the appropriate use of health care resources for the very aged and terminally ill and the possible substitution of nursing home, hospice, or home health care for more expensive hospital admissions.[12,13]

Changes are now occurring in utilization rates as a result of recent policy initiatives. There has been a major increase in the use of the Medicare home health benefit since 1981 (see Chapter 8), and hospital use has declined. Even before the introduction of prospective payment for Medicare hospital admissions in October 1983, the average length of stay had declined. Recent data show that there was a further 9.7-percent decline in average length of stay for Medicare patients between 1983 and 1984 and a 3.5-percent decline in the number of admissions per 1,000 enrollees.[14] Age-specific data on changes in utilization rates are not available at the time of writing.

Medicaid: Utilization and Expenditures

The Medicaid program has had an eleven-fold increase in expenditures between 1967 and 1983, from $2.9 to over $34 billion (see Table 5-11). Over 75 percent of these expenditures were distributed almost equally between acute hospital and nursing home care.

Even with population increases and changes in the age structure, the number of Medicaid recipients has remained almost constant over time, with a slight downward trend since 1977 (see Table 5-12). Physician services and prescription drugs are the services provided to the highest proportion of Medicaid recipients. On the other hand, as shown in Table 5-13, the highest vendor payments in 1983 were for all types of nursing home care; intermediate care facilities received a higher proportion of payments than skilled nursing facilities.

Table 5-14 shows the percentage of Medicaid recipients aged 65 and over as a percentage of total recipients, by state, from 1975 to 1983. Although the national average is 15 percent, the proportions vary considerably and do not correlate with the percentage of the state population aged 65 and over. In Texas the elderly constitute more than 30 percent of Medicaid recipients, but only 9.6 percent of the state population is in this age group. In New Jersey the elderly represent only 9.8 percent of the Medicaid population, even though 11.7 percent of the state population is aged 65 and over.

Table 5-11. Medicaid expenditures and percentage distribution by type of service, selected years 1967-1983.

Type of service	Year						
	1967	1970	1975	1979	1980	1981	1983
Total	\$2.9	\$5.2	\$13.5	\$21.8	\$25.5	\$29.0	\$34.0
				Amount in billions			
				Percentage			
All services	100.0	100.0	100.0	100.0	100.0	100.0	100.0
Hospital care	42.3	42.9	34.6	37.3	36.7	36.3	39.9
Physician services	10.9	13.3	14.0	10.1	9.8	9.9	8.7
Dentist services	4.4	3.2	2.9	1.8	2.0	2.1	1.4
Other professional services	0.9	1.4	1.5	2.3	2.0	1.7	2.3
Drugs and drug sundries	7.2	7.9	6.6	5.5	5.5	5.5	5.5
Nursing home care	31.7	27.2	36.0	39.6	39.8	39.7	36.4
Other health services*	2.6	4.1	4.4	3.2	4.3	4.8	5.8

* Other services include laboratory and radiological services, home health, and family planning services.

Source: National Center for Health Statistics: Health, United States, 1984. DHHS Pub. No. (PHS)84-1232, Public Health Service. Washington, D.C., U.S. Government Printing Office, December 1984.

Table 5-12. Unduplicated number of recipients under Medicaid by selected medical services, 1972 - 1983.

Recipients in thousands

Fiscal year	Total	Inpatient services in general hospital	Skilled nursing facility services	ICF services Mentally retarded	ICF services All other	Inpatient services in mental hospital	Physician services	Home health services
Ending June:								
1972	17,606	2,832	552	-	-	40	12,282	105
1973	19,622	3,256	678	29	433	77	13,278	110
1974	21,462	3,291	661	39	588	72	14,970	144
1975	21,958	3,431	628	68	681	67	15,179	343
1976	22,766	3,550	635	88	723	82	15,604	319
Ending September:								
1977	22,753	3,766	639	107	753	84	16,053	371
1978	21,918	3,781	637	103	739	76	15,648	376
1979	21,520	3,606	608	114	765	74	15,147	359
1980	21,605	3,680	609	121	789	66	13,765	392
1981	21,980	3,703	623	151	762	90	14,403	401
1982	21,603	3,530	559	149	765	72	13,894	377
1983	21,471	3,659	573	145	792	82	14,022	419

Percentage change

Ending June:								
1973	11.5	15.0	22.8	–	–	92.5	8.1	4.8
1974	9.4	1.1	-2.5	34.4	35.8	-6.5	12.7	30.9
1975	2.3	4.3	-5.0	74.4	15.8	-6.9	1.4	138.2
1976	3.7	3.5	1.1	29.4	6.2	22.4	2.8	-7.0
Ending September:								
1977	-0.1	6.1	0.6	21.6	4.1	2.4	2.9	16.3
1978	-3.7	0.4	-0.3	-3.7	-1.9	-9.5	-2.5	1.3
1979	-1.8	-4.6	-4.6	10.7	3.5	-2.6	-3.2	-4.5
1980	0.4	2.1	0.2	6.1	3.1	-10.8	-9.1	9.2
1981	1.7	0.6	2.3	24.8	-3.4	36.4	4.6	2.3
1982	-1.7	-4.7	-10.3	-1.3	0.4	-20.0	-3.5	-6.0
1983	-0.6	3.7	2.5	-2.7	3.5	13.9	0.9	11.1

* 1983 data are preliminary figures.

Source: Office of Financial and Actuarial Analysis, Bureau of Data Management and Strategy, Health Care Financing Administration, 1984.

Table 5-13. Medicaid vendor payments by type of medical service, 1972-1983.

Fiscal year	Total	Inpatient services in general hospital	Skilled nursing facility services	ICF Services		Inpatient services in mental hospital	Physician services	Home health services
				Mentally retarded	All other			
				Amount in millions				
Ending June:								
1972	$6,300	$2,557	$1,471	$ -	$ -	$113	$794	$24
1973	8,639	2,660	1,959	165	895	349	926	25
1974	9,983	2,887	2,002	203	1,381	406	1,083	31
1975	12,242	3,374	2,434	380	1,885	405	1,225	70
1976	14,091	3,904	2,476	635	2,209	529	1,369	134
Ending September:								
1977	16,239	4,562	2,691	917	2,637	586	1,505	180
1978	17,992	4,992	3,125	1,192	3,104	665	1,554	210
1979	20,472	5,655	3,379	1,488	3,773	778	1,625	263
1980	23,311	6,412	3,685	1,989	4,202	775	1,875	332
1981	27,204	7,194	4,035	2,996	4,507	877	2,101	428
1982	29,399	7,670	4,427	3,467	4,979	974	2,086	496
1983	32,316	8,782	4,621	3,866	5,380	976	2,173	597

Percentage change

Ending June:								
1973	37.1	4.0	33.2	–	–	208.9	16.6	4.2
1974	15.6	8.5	2.2	23.0	54.3	16.3	17.0	24.0
1975	22.6	16.9	21.6	87.2	36.5	-0.2	13.1	125.8
1976	15.1	15.7	1.7	67.1	17.2	30.6	11.8	91.4
Ending September:								
1977	15.2	16.9	8.7	44.4	19.4	10.8	9.9	34.3
1978	10.8	9.4	16.1	30.0	17.7	13.5	3.3	16.7
1979	13.8	13.3	8.1	24.8	21.6	17.0	5.2	25.2
1980	13.9	13.4	9.1	33.7	11.4	-0.4	14.7	26.2
1981	16.7	12.2	9.5	50.6	7.3	13.2	12.1	28.9
1982	8.1	6.6	9.7	15.7	10.5	11.1	-0.7	15.9
1983	9.9	14.5	4.4	11.5	8.1	0.2	4.2	20.4

* 1983 data are preliminary.

Source: Office of Financial and Actuarial Analysis, Bureau of Data Management and Strategy, Health Care Financing Administration, 1984.

Table 5-14. Medicaid recipients aged 65 and over as a percentage of total recipients, by state, 1975, 1977, 1979, 1981, 1983.

	Percentage aged 65 and over				
	1975	1977	1979	1981	1983
United States	16.4	15.3	15.6	15.3	15.1
Alabama	37.3	34.5	29.9	29.7	27.8
Alaska	10.9	10.4	13.3	14.7	11.1
Arizona					
Arkansas	39.1	30.4	29.6	27.5	28.5
California	19.1	16.7	15.6	15.7	16.0
Colorado	21.1	19.7	21.2	25.5	25.3
Connecticut	12.6	27.4	12.8	15.9	14.8
Delaware	9.0	7.6	8.0	9.9	10.6
District of Columbia	7.9	8.8	8.5	9.5	10.2
Florida	22.3	22.2	26.1	21.6	19.8
Georgia	21.9	28.6	25.1	23.9	20.3
Hawaii	8.7	10.2	10.6	11.6	12.6
Idaho	15.7	15.6	16.1	16.0	16.7
Illinois	6.7	7.7	8.1	7.6	7.8
Indiana	13.9	13.2	14.3	15.6	13.8
Iowa	20.6	19.6	19.7	16.6	15.6
Kansas	14.3	13.6	15.1	17.9	16.6
Kentucky	21.7	16.4	18.0	15.7	15.3
Louisiana	32.0	30.7	27.3	24.0	25.6
Maine	16.9	15.3	16.2	16.0	17.0
Maryland	13.1	14.4	12.8	12.0	11.4
Massachusetts	22.3	20.0	20.0	16.6	24.0
Michigan	11.2	10.2	10.1	9.7	7.4
Minnesota	18.5	18.6	18.6	16.6	15.9
Mississippi	29.8	29.5	28.5	22.6	22.5
Missouri	24.9	19.9	20.9	20.3	19.2
Montana	17.0	18.1	17.7	15.1	16.8
Nebraska	22.3	22.6	22.3	20.1	17.4
Nevada	18.0	19.2	23.2	22.4	22.2
New Hampshire	21.7	20.5	21.2	21.9	22.2
New Jersey	9.2	9.2	9.2	9.4	9.8
New Mexico	13.4	14.4	13.7	13.4	14.2
New York	13.7	13.7	13.7	15.8	16.1
North Carolina	27.6	21.6	22.1	20.0	23.8
North Dakota	24.3	24.0	25.5	30.9	34.6
Ohio	14.8	14.8	14.8	10.6	10.0
Oklahoma	27.1	26.6	21.3	19.5	24.6
Oregon	10.6	10.7	8.7	10.9	14.0
Pennsylvania	7.7	6.8	7.8	11.5	11.2
Rhode Island	19.5	25.3	25.6	18.7	19.8
South Carolina	31.8	23.7	23.4	18.3	19.9
South Dakota	27.5	24.3	23.6	25.6	25.3
Tennessee	26.3	24.8	25.9	22.7	21.7
Texas	34.0	36.3	35.6	34.2	33.0
Utah	10.1	10.8	14.2	11.3	21.9
Vermont	17.6	15.2	17.3	14.8	14.3
Virginia	19.3	19.4	19.8	19.7	20.2
Washington	13.7	15.3	15.0	14.9	15.1
West Virginia	16.4	17.3	27.3	15.8	14.1
Wisconsin	22.9	20.4	18.2	15.0	13.9
Wyoming	17.6	17.5	16.1	17.5	18.1

Source: Office of Financial and Actuarial Analysis, Division of Medical Cost Estimates, Medical Statistics Branch, Health Care Financing Administration, 1983.

This is indicative of the ability of individual states to determine eligibility for Medicaid services. States electing to extend coverage to the "medically needy" enable a high proportion of their nursing home population to be eligible for Medicaid, having depleted their resources or transferred assets. It has been estimated that nursing home services, including psychiatric hospitals for the elderly, constituted 71 percent of Medicaid expenditures for those aged 65 and over in 1981.[15]

Medicaid-reimbursed long-term care services are not used solely by the elderly, however. Intermediate care facilities for the mentally retarded (ICFMR) have been the most rapidly growing Medicaid benefit in recent years.[2] The second-highest growth has been in home health care services (see Table 5-13).

Recipients of Both Medicare and Medicaid

A comparison of the characteristics of those eligible for both Medicare and Medicaid with those enrolled in Medicare alone, using 1978 data, demonstrated a strong interrelationship between the two programs.[5] In terms of demographic characteristics, those entitled to both Medicare and Medicaid were shown to be relatively older than the Medicare-only population, with a mean age of 76.6 compared with 73.6 for the Medicare-only population, and to have a much higher proportion of women (71 percent compared with 59 percent); also, although 75 percent of dual eligibles were white, there was a higher proportion of minority races in this group than in the general population.[5]

The proportion of those who received Medicare benefits was considerably higher for the dual eligibles than for the Medicare-only population, with higher average reimbursements under both HI and SMI. There was also considerable excess mortality for those with both Medicare and Medicaid in the 65 to 69 age group compared with the Medicare-only population, but the differences in mortality experience declined with age, so that there was no difference in mortality rates for those aged 80 and over.[5]

These findings, which show the elderly poor to have high utilization rates of health care services, indicate that restriction of benefits under one program could have a substantial impact on the other. If hospital services were restricted under Medicare or cost sharing were increased, the increase would be shifted to Medicaid; if Medicaid long-term care services were restricted, there could be an increase in acute hospital care utilization.[5]

Private Health Insurance

The size of the private health insurance industry, including Blue Cross and Blue Shield, commercial insurance, and prepaid and self-insured plans, has grown steadily over the years, so that in 1983 53 percent of private expenditures for personal health care were reimbursed by private insurance. Health insurance premiums have been growing at 14 percent per year since 1950 compared with an average 11-percent increase in personal health care expenditures.[2] Eighty-four percent of the population under age 65 had some form of private health insurance coverage in 1982.[16]

Many individuals aged 65 and over purchase private health insurance to supplement Medicare. Those purchasing this "medigap" insurance may not fully comprehend the insurance limitations; the main function of the policies is to provide "first dollar" coverage of deductibles and coinsurance payments. The insurance is the same as for Medicare with respect to coverage and length of stay, nursing home benefits are generally confined to posthospital skilled nursing care, and "medigap" offers little protection against the financial consequences of catastrophic illness.[10]

In 1977 it was estimated that 65.2 percent of the elderly were covered by Medicare and private insurance, 10.6 percent had both Medicare and Medicaid, 20.4 percent had Medicare alone, and a further 3.8 percent were either uninsured or had other coverage under the Veterans Administration.[6] Health insurance industry data show that 59 percent of the Medicare population aged 65 and over had private health insurance in 1982, so there has been an apparent decline.[16] It is now estimated that 13 to 14 percent of the elderly are covered by both Medicare and Medicaid.[5,10]

The 1977 survey also demonstrated that only 60 percent of those aged 75 and over had Medicare and private insurance compared with 70 percent of those aged 65 to 69, only 31 percent of minority races had insurance compared with 69 percent of whites, and those with both low income and poor health also had lower coverage rates.[6] In 1977 premiums for Part B of Medicare amounted to about $90 per year, and the mean cost of private insurance for Medicare beneficiaries was an additional $304.[6]

Medigap policies are projected to have covered 7 percent of total health care expenditures for the elderly in 1984.[10]

As far as insurance for long-term care is concerned, even though there has been some conceptual work on the subject,[17] the private medical insurance market is at an early stage of development. Benefits have been mainly restricted to limited coverage for nursing home services, but home care is now being added to some policies in order to promote private long-term care insurance.

Out-of-Pocket Expenditures

Direct payments for health care have declined as a percentage of total health expenditures for all age groups in recent years, from 52 percent in

1965 to 27 percent in 1983 (see Table 5-2). The decline has been greater for the elderly than for other age groups; the elderly were responsible for 29 percent of personal health care expenditures in 1977, but only 25 percent in 1984.[10] On the other hand, because of inflation in health care costs and increases in Medicare copayments, out-of-pocket expenditures have recently begun to increase as a percentage of annual income for the elderly.

While individual liability for the costs of acute hospital care has shown a major decline, nursing home care continues to represent the biggest out-of-pocket liability for the elderly: 50 percent in 1977 and 52 percent in 1984.[3,10]

In 1966, before the introduction of Medicare, the elderly were paying 15 percent of their annual income for out-of-pocket health expenditures.[18] As shown in Table 5-15, out-of-pocket expenditures represented 12 percent of mean income in 1977 and were estimated to be nearly 15 percent in 1984, rising to 18 percent by 1989.[18]

The limitations of these data are that they do not reflect the out-of-pocket expenses for the average noninstitutionalized Medicare beneficiary in that the estimates do not include the cost of health insurance premiums for SMI or private insurance but do include direct payments for nursing home care.

Table 5-15. Personal health care expenditures for individuals aged 65 and over, 1977, 1980, 1984, 1989*

	Per capita health care expenditures			
Source of funds	1977	1980	1984	1989
Total	$1,785	$2,515	$4,256	$6,637
Private	719	976	1,543	2,433
Consumer	712	966	1,526	2,409
Out-of-pocket	522	721	1,072	1,705
Insurance	115	148	308	509
Medicare premiums	75	96	146	195
Other private	7	10	17	24
Government	1,066	1,540	2,713	4,204
Medicare	713	1,061	1,931	3,057
Medicaid	249	333	543	807
Other government	104	146	239	340

* Data derived from the Bureau of the Census, and the Health Care Financing Administration, July 1984.

Source: Select Committee on Aging, U.S. House of Representatives, Fact Sheet, October 1984.

Table 5-16. Median out-of-pocket charges and mean percentage of charges and of family income that was made out-of-pocket, by selected characteristics, 1980.

Characteristic	Median out-of-of-pocket charge	Estimated population with expenditures (In thousands)	Mean percentage of charges	Mean percentage of income
Total	$156	20,869	56.67	5.58
Age				
65-74	143	13,481	57.17	4.91
75-84	188	6,227	56.71	7.27
85 & over	129	1,161	50.67	4.38
Sex				
Male	137	8,113	55.02	4.7
Female	173	12,756	57.72	6.14
Race				
White	165	18,930	57.62	5.07
All other	75	1,939	47.45	10.57
Region				
Northeast	138	3,948	56.81	9.4
North Central	161	5,137	61.14	3.84
South	180	7,106	57.13	5.47
West	130	4,679	50.95	4.42
Family income in 1980				
Under $5,000	126	4,805	52.72	14.41
$5,000-$7,999	166	2,821	59.19	4.61
$8,000-$9,999	161	3,743	58.73	4.58
$10,000-$14,999	163	3,967	56.78	2.54
$15,000-$24,999	165	3,367	55.45	1.86
$25,000 or more	158	2,167	60.28	0.81
Poverty status in 1980				
Below poverty level	116	4,241	52.85	14.83
100-149 percent	176	4,407	55.81	5.1
150-199 percent	153	3,759	60.19	3.64
200-299 percent	158	4,182	54.32	2.83
300 percent or more	178	4,279	60.54	1.53

Source: Kovar M.G., Expenditures for the medical care of elderly people living in the community throughout 1980. National Medical Care Utilization and Expenditure Survey, Data Report No. 4, DHHS Pub. No. (PHS)84-20000, National Center for Health Statistics, Public Health Service. Washington, D.C., U.S. Government Printing Office, November 1983.

Table 5-17. Personal health care expenditures as a percentage of income for individuals aged 65 and over in 1977, 1980, 1984 and 1989*

Elderly consumer costs as a percentage of income	1977	1980	1984	1989
Percentage of mean income	12.3	12.68	14.52	18.4
Percentage of median income	18.46	18.53	21.4	-

* Derived from data from the Bureau of the Census, the Health Care Financing Administration and the Bureau of Labor Statistics, July 1984.

Source: Select Committee on Aging, U.S. House of Representatives, Fact Sheet, October 1984.

Results from a 1980 survey of the elderly noninstitutionalized population are shown in Table 5-16. These data indicate that on average, out-of-pocket charges for medical care amounted to 15 percent of the 1980 family income for elderly people below the poverty level, but only 2 percent of the 1980 family income for elderly people at 300 percent of the poverty level or above. Expenditures for the care of nursing home patients and payments for health insurance premiums and over-the-counter drugs are not included in these estimates.[7]

Table 5-17 shows the actual and projected personal health care expenditures for the elderly for 1977, 1980, 1984, and 1989. It is projected that the elderly will assume a much greater responsibility for their own care between 1984 and 1989.[8,18]

Summary

Although national health care expenditures have been increasing constantly as a proportion of GNP since 1929, the rate of increase accelerated after the introduction of the Medicare and Medicaid programs in 1966. There was a major increase in the proportion of public, and specifically federal, funding of health care with a commensurate decline in the proportion of private funding. Since then, federal expenditures, particularly for the Medicare program, have increased at a far higher rate than state or private health care expenditures, although all have grown substantially.

Almost the entire elderly population is eligible for federally subsidized health insurance under Medicare which, in 1972, was extended to cover younger, eligible disabled persons. Coverage is predominantly for the costs associated with an acute episode of illness, and over 90 percent of Medicare expenditures are for acute hospital and physician services.

Medicaid is a joint federal-state program; federal grants match state expenditures based on a formula related to the per capita income of the state. The program provides access to a wide range of medical care, for certain low-income groups, including the elderly, a high proportion of which is for long-term care in nursing homes. States have considerable discretion in determining both eligibility and range of service provision under the Medicaid program. As a result, the total number of Medicaid recipients has remained almost constant over time, and state expenditures for health care represent the same proportion of total health care costs as before the introduction of the program. In most states a disproportionate percentage of Medicaid recipients are elderly and are eligible for both Medicare and Medicaid.

The spiraling costs of the Medicare program have led to recent initiatives to restrict payments made under the open-ended reimbursement system. The unanticipated growth in the elderly population, including the extreme aged, has clearly contributed to the high rate of increase in federal Medicare expenditures; however, data showing the variation by state in per capita utilization rates and expenditures, the high proportion of payments being made for individuals in the last year of life, and the high use of hospitals as opposed to nursing home or community-based alternatives have all indicated that measures could be introduced to improve efficiency and restrain total Medicare costs.

Changes that have been instituted in the interests of cost containment in the Medicare program include: liberalization of the home health benefit, prospective payment for acute hospital care, with the objective of achieving more efficient management of hospital admissions, and a temporary freeze on physician reimbursement. Preliminary data show that there have been recent reductions in length of hospital stay and in the rate of admission for Medicare patients, with the fastest growing sectors of the Medicare budget being for home health and hospital outpatient care. The effects of providing increased access to more comprehensive pre-paid health care benefits in health maintenance organizations have not yet been assessed.

In addition to restrictions on reimbursements to health care providers, there have been substantial increases in copayments and deductibles to beneficiaries. A high proportion of the elderly purchase private health insurance to supplement Medicare benefits. In general, the "medigap" policies provide "first dollar" coverage for Medicare deductibles and coinsurance but do not afford protection against the costs of catastrophic illness or long-term care.

Even excluding the costs of the premiums for private insurance coverage, out-of-pocket expenditures by individuals now account for the same proportion of elderly income as before the introduction of Medicare, with the highest percentage being paid by those with the lowest incomes. It is predicted that the elderly will be required to assume responsibility for an increasing proportion of health care costs. The result may be an increase in the percentage of elderly persons eligible for both Medicare and Medicaid.

Those dually eligible for Medicare and Medicaid tend to be older than the Medicare-only population, to have a high proportion of women and minorities, and to be in poorer health. For these individuals there is an association between care provided under the two programs, with Medicare being the primary payor for Medicare-covered services. Restrictions on the Medicare benefit could result in cost shifting to Medicaid, and vice versa.

REFERENCES

1. Stevens R. American Medicine and the Public Interest. New Haven and London, Yale University Press, 1971.
2. Gibson R. M., Levit K. R., Lazenby H., Waldo D. R. National health care expenditures, 1983. Health Care Financing Review 6: 2: 1–29, 1984.
3. Fisher C. R. Differences by age groups in health care spending. Health Care Financing Review 1: 4: 65–90, 1980.
4. The Medicare and Medicaid Data Book, 1983. Health Care Financing Administration, HCFA Pub No 03156, December 1983.
5. McMillan A., Pine P. L., Gornick M., Prihoda R. A study of the 'crossover population': aged persons entitled to both Medicare and Medicaid. Health Care Financing Review 4: 4: 19–43, 1983.
6. Cafferata G. L. Private health insurance coverage of the Medicare population, National Health Care Expenditures Study, Data Preview 18, DHHS Pub. No. (PHS)84-3362, National Center for Health Services Research, September, 1984.
7. Kovar M. G. Expenditures for the medical care of elderly people living in the community throughout 1980. National Medical Care Utilization and Expenditure Survey, Data Report No. 4, DHHS Pub. No. (PHS)84-20000, National Center for Health Statistics, Public Health Service, Washington, D.C. U.S. Government Printing Office, November 1983.
8. Freeland M. S., Schendler C. E. National health expenditure growth in the 1980's: an aging population, new technologies and increasing competition. Health Care Financing Review 4: 3: 1–58, 1983.
9. Levit K. R. Personal health care expenditures by state, selected years, 1966–1978. Health Care Financing Review 4: 2: 1–45, 1982.
10. Waldo D., Lazenby H. C. Demographic characteristics and health care use and expenditures by the aged in the United States: 1977–1984. Health Care Financing Review 6: 1: 1–29, 1984.
11. Lubitz J., Deacon R. The rise in the incidence of hospitalizations for the aged, 1967 to 1979. Health Care Financing Review 3: 3: 21–40, 1982.
12. National Center for Health Statistics. Lubitz J., Prihoda, R. Use and costs of Medicare services in the last years of life. Health, United States 1983. DHHS Pub. No. (PHS)84-1232, Public Health Service, Washington, D.C. U.S. Government Printing Office, December 1983.

13. Young K. M., Fisher C. R. Medicare episodes of illness: a study of hospital, skilled nursing facility and home health agency care. Health Care Financing Review 2: 2: 1–23, 1980.
14. Health Care Financing Administration, Bureau of Data Management and Strategy. Health Care Spending Bulletin, No. 85-02, April 1985.
15. Macken C. L. 1982 Long-Term Care Survey: national estimates of functional impairments among the elderly living in the community. Office of Research and Demonstrations, Health Care Financing Administration, (working paper), 1984.
16. Source Book of Health Insurance Data, 1982–1983. Health Insurance Association of America, 1984.
17. Meiners M. R. The case for long-term care insurance. Health Affairs 2: 2: 55–77, 1983.
18. House Select Committee on Aging, Fact Sheet, October 11, 1984

6

Nursing Homes

To many legislators, administrators, and others, nursing home care is synonymous with long-term care.

The origins of the nursing home industry lie in the poorhouses and almshouses of the 19th and early 20th centuries in the "homes for the aged" established by voluntary and religious organizations and in small proprietary boarding houses that provided lodging for the elderly and where the line between the provision of "hotel" services and personal and nursing care for those in declining health was not clearly delineated. By the 1940's, as hospitals became increasingly specialized in the treatment of acute illness, they also began to construct separate nursing home facilities. This trend was later encouraged by the Hill Burton Act.

Apart from demographic changes, the major developments in the nursing home industry since the 1930's have resulted from three types of legislation that provided:

- Income maintenance to aged and disabled persons, enabling them to purchase nursing home care.
- Loans and grants to build and improve nursing home facilities.
- Direct payment to providers for the cost of nursing home services on behalf of residents.[1]

Income Maintenance Legislation

The Social Security Act of 1935 mandated a program of Old Age Assistance (OAA) with eligibility and means-tested benefits determined by the states, but with payment specifically forbidden to the "inmates of public institutions."[2] This led to the virtual demise of the local "poorhouses," which had poor reputations and stigmatized the inmates, and to the expansion of proprietary nursing homes as the elderly were enabled to pay for care. In 1950 Aid to the Disabled (AD), which was similar to OAA, became available, and assistance was extended to the inmates of public institutions, so that some former poorhouses have survived as publicly operated nursing homes.

113

Under the 1972 Social Security Amendments, the OAA and AD programs were abolished and replaced by the federally financed and administered Supplementary Security Income (SSI) program (see Chapter 3).

Legislation to Increase the Stock of Nursing Homes

The demand for nursing home care grew in the 1940's and 1950's as the number of elderly and their ability to pay for care increased. The resulting shortage of facilities led to legislation to increase the supply.

The 1946 Hill Burton Act provided grants, loans, and loan guarantees to nonprofit and government hospitals for construction and modernization where additional facilities were needed in the community. In 1954 financial support was extended to nonprofit and government nursing homes, also to be based on established need. Assistance was limited to homes capable of providing a high level of skilled nursing care.

Hill Burton funding had a significant effect on the development of the voluntary nonprofit sector of the nursing home industry. Lobbying by the proprietary nursing home industry in the 1950's led to loans being made available for construction, expansion, equipment, supplies, and working capital from the Small Business Administration in 1956. This did not satisfy the demands of the industry; in 1959 mortgage insurance for proprietary nursing homes was channeled through the Federal Housing Administration, under Section 232 of the Housing Act, if a "certificate of need" had been issued by the appropriate state agency. Additional funding in rural areas has come from the Farmers Home Administration of the Department of Agriculture and through the Appalachian Regional Development Act of 1965.[1]

"Vendor Payment" Legislation

From the beginning of the OAA and AD programs, funds were available for nursing home and other medical care. At first the cost of care was paid to the recipient, who then reimbursed the provider of service. Amendments in 1950 to the Social Security Act permitted welfare agencies to make direct "medical vendor payments" to the providers on behalf of the aged and disabled recipients. States had the right to determine the income level at which eligibility began, and two methods were adopted: the "in or out" system under which only those whose income fell below the specified level were eligible for either money payments or medical care, and the "spend-down" system under which those who were ineligible for money payments could become eligible for medical vendor payments if their expenses were high enough to bring net income down to eligibility levels. The high cost of nursing home care meant that many individuals in the "spend-down" states who were not eligible for money payments qualified for nursing home care.

Most states reimbursed on a flat-rate basis; some required nursing homes to accept the reimbursement as full payment, and others permitted the home to charge a supplemental amount to the resident or family. The 1950 amendments mandated that states introduce licensure for those homes to which vendor payments were made.[1]

Medical Assistance for the Aged

This program, enacted in 1960, ran only until Medicare and Medicaid were implemented in 1966. It was essentially an extension of the OAA vendor payment program, but it permitted states to provide coverage for the "medically indigent" and had open-ended federal contributions of 50 to 80 percent of the cost, depending on the per capita income of the state. By 1965 about 300,000 individuals were receiving nursing home care under the program, a significant increase from preprogram levels.[1,2]

Medicare and Medicaid

While other legislation may have had measurable effects on the development of the nursing home industry, the introduction of the Medicare and Medicaid nursing home benefits in 1967 provided the major impetus to growth.

Medicare introduced the concept of the "extended care facility" to provide posthospital skilled nursing care in nursing homes or rehabilitation institutions as a less expensive alternative to lengthy hospitalization.[3] Medicare-reimbursed nursing home care must be preceded by a hospital stay of at least three days. Under the 1982 Tax Equity and Fiscal Responsibility Act, legislation was passed to allow this provision to be eliminated at such time that it is determined that the measure will not lead to increased costs. Currently, the change has not been implemented.

The Medicaid program was introduced to provide medical care, including "skilled nursing home" care, to all those eligible for cash assistance programs and to others determined by each state to be "medically indigent." Prior hospitalization was never required, and providers of service have been required to accept the Medicaid payment as payment in full. Within a year of the introduction of Medicaid, amendments were passed in an attempt to reduce costs; among them was the designation of a new classification of nursing homes—intermediate care facilities (ICF's)—to provide care between the skilled nursing home and room and board services.

In 1972, under amendments to the Social Security Act, "extended care facilities" under Medicare were combined with "skilled nursing homes" under Medicaid into a new classification of "skilled nursing facilities" (SNF's).[1] More nursing hours per day are required in skilled than intermediate facilities, and SNF status makes a facility potentially eligible for Medicare and ensures higher Medicaid reimbursements.

All Medicare-reimbursed patients and a very high proportion of private patients are in SNF's; generally ICF's serve only the Medicaid population, but the Medicaid program has become the major source of public funding for long-term care in the United States, while only a very small proportion of Medicare reimbursements are for nursing home care (see below).

DATA SOURCES

Sources of information for the tables presented in this chapter are as follows.

The main data sources regarding developments and trends in nursing home care are from the National Master Facility Inventories (NMFI) and the National Nursing Home Surveys (NNHS), both carried out by the National Center for Health Statistics.

The NMFI's are censuses of selected characteristics of "nursing and related care homes," including size, ownership and staffing levels. Data have been published for 1963, 1967, 1969, 1971, 1973, 1976, 1978, and 1980.[4-12] At the time of writing, findings from the 1982 MFI had not yet been published. Data from the NMFI are not necessarily comparable over time, because the criteria for inclusion change, and certain types of facilities are added and others excluded (see below).

National Nursing Home Surveys were undertaken in 1963, 1964, 1969, 1973–1974, and 1977.[13-17] These are nationwide sample surveys of nursing homes, resident characteristics, discharges, and staffing levels. The latest survey was carried out in 1985.

The Medicare/Medicaid Automated Certification System (MMACS), implemented by the Health Standards and Quality Bureau of the Health Care Financing Administration, collects data relating to all facilities certified under Medicare and/or Medicaid. These data include all certified hospital-based nursing home units.

Data on expenditures for nursing home care under Medicare and Medicaid are available from the Division of Medical Cost Estimates of the Health Care Financing Administration.

Nursing Home and Bed Supply

The first Master Facility Inventory was carried out in 1963 and the second in 1967, a year after the introduction of Medicare and Medicaid. While the number of nursing homes increased by 2,440, or 15 percent, between 1963 and 1967, the number of beds increased by 47 percent, raising the average number of beds per home by ten (see Table 6-1). There

Table 6-1. Number of nursing homes and beds, percentage change and average bed size of homes, 1963, 1967, 1969, 1971, 1973, 1976, 1980 and 1982.

Year	Homes	Percentage change	Beds	Percentage change	Average bed size
1982	26,175	7.0	1,508,732	4.0	63
1980	23,065	13.0	1,537,338	9.0	67
1976	20,468	-6.0	1,414,865	7.0	69
1973	21,834	-1.0	1,327,704	10.0	61
1971	22,004	16.0	1,201,598	27.0	55
1969	18,910	-1.0	943,876	13.0	50
1967	19,141	15.0	836,554	47.0	44
1963	16,701		568,560	-	34

Source: National Center for Health Statistics: Master Facility Inventories, 1963, 1967, 1969, 1971, 1973, 1976, 1980, 1982.

was a further 30-percent increase in the number of beds between 1967 and 1971, but the rate of increase declined in the 1970's, to 26 percent overall from 1971 to 1980.[4-11]

Although the number of beds increased with every MFI from 1963 to 1980, and the average bed size of homes increased progressively up to 1976, the actual number of homes has fluctuated, with a net decline shown in some time periods. This is because of the changing criteria used for the inclusion of nursing and related care homes in the MFI. Since 1978, for example, many small facilities such as homes for the deaf, blind, and emotionally disturbed have been excluded, and in 1980 hospital-based nursing homes were excluded because of difficulty in obtaining comprehensive data. On the other hand, over 2,500 adult foster care homes in Michigan and 1,000 community care homes in California were identified as meeting the definitional requirements for inclusion in 1980.[11]

Preliminary data from the 1982 MFI show an overall increase of 7 percent in the number of beds between 1980 and 1982, but 50 percent of this increase (52,032 of 104,662) is accounted for by an increase in community care beds, mainly in small facilities in California. The increase in actual nursing home beds was only 4 percent.[18]

Table 6-2 shows the relationship between nursing homes and the number of nursing home beds, as recorded in the 1980 MFI, and the population aged 65 and over. The average number of beds per 1,000 persons aged 65 and over varies greatly by state. The states with the highest average number—South Dakota (95.0), Nebraska (92.2), and Washington (90.8)—had four times as many as those with the lowest average—Florida (21.4), New Mexico (26.5), and West Virginia (27.0).

In view of the fact that small nursing homes go in and out of business more frequently than others and meet criteria for inclusion in the NMFI

Table 6-2. Number of persons 65 years and over, nursing and related care homes, beds, beds per 1,000 population aged 65 and over, and rank, by state, 1980.

State	Population 65 & over (Thousands)	Homes	Beds	Beds per 1,000 population 65 & over	Rank
United States	25,544	23,065	1,537,338	60.2	-
Alabama	440	210	20,651	46.9	37
Alaska	12	9	1,029	85.8	8
Arizona	307	120	9,309	30.3	48
Arkansas	312	196	19,238	61.7	26
California	2,415	4,134	163,482	67.7	21
Colorado	247	161	17,310	70.0	19
Connecticut	365	320	21,244	58.2	27
Delaware	59	32	2,530	42.9	42
District of Columbia	74	49	3,180	43.0	41
Florida	1,685	355	36,122	21.4	51
Georgia	517	326	30,041	58.1	28
Hawaii	76	243	2,805	36.9	46
Idaho	94	57	4,355	46.3	38
Illinois	1,261	761	88,383	70.1	18
Indiana	585	458	44,511	76.1	13
Iowa	387	489	34,641	89.5	4
Kansas	306	357	25,208	82.4	9
Kentucky	410	310	26,265	64.1	25
Louisiana	404	201	21,672	53.6	31
Maine	141	424	11,317	80.3	12
Maryland	396	187	20,726	52.3	33
Massachusetts	727	800	52,254	71.9	17
Michigan	912	3,038	80,082	87.8	6
Minnesota	480	409	41,931	87.4	7
Mississippi	289	156	12,253	42.4	43
Missouri	648	867	46,691	72.1	15
Montana	85	86	5,652	66.5	22
Nebraska	206	262	18,990	92.2	2
Nevada	66	31	2,022	30.6	47
New Hampshire	103	87	6,672	64.8	24
New Jersey	860	471	37,825	44.0	40
New Mexico	116	72	3,075	26.5	50
New York	2,161	828	103,952	48.1	35
North Carolina	602	940	32,173	53.4	32
North Dakota	80	86	6,450	80.6	11
Ohio	1,169	960	76,280	65.3	23
Oklahoma	376	348	27,101	72.1	16
Oregon	303	196	17,382	57.4	29
Pennsylvania	1,531	550	75,907	49.6	34
Rhode Island	127	110	8,653	68.1	20
South Carolina	287	194	11,990	41.8	45
South Dakota	91	138	8,647	95.0	1
Tennessee	518	249	21,692	41.9	44
Texas	1,371	997	101,328	73.9	14
Utah	109	74	5,052	46.3	39
Vermont	58	172	4,706	81.1	10
Virginia	505	436	27,377	54.2	30
Washington	431	543	39,153	90.8	3
West Virginia	238	120	6,423	27.0	49
Wisconsin	564	427	49,847	88.4	5
Wyoming	37	19	1,759	47.5	36

Source: National Center for Health Statistics: Nursing and related care homes as reported from the 1980 NMFI Survey. Vital and Health Statistics, Series 14 No. 29. DHHS Pub. No. (PHS)84-1824, Public Health Service. Washington, D.C., U.S. Government Printing Office, December 1983.

one year and not the next, it has been recommended that in comparing trends over time, only those facilities with 25 or more beds should be included.[12]

For homes with 25 or more beds, the average number of beds per 1,000 population aged 65 and over increased by 24 percent, from 43.4 to 56.8 between 1969 and 1973, but has remained almost constant since that time despite the increase in the proportion of the elderly population aged 75 and over and 85 and over that has characterized the period (see Table 6-3). Some states, such as Michigan, have shown an increase in each time period; others, such as Wisconsin, had major increases between 1969 and 1973 followed by a relative decline.

Ownership, Bed Size, and Staffing Levels

Although the trend, as shown in Table 6-1, has been to increasing average bed size, in 1980 one half of all nursing homes included in the MFI had fewer than 50 beds, while 40 percent of all beds were in homes with 100 to 199 beds.[11]

In 1967 78 percent of nursing homes were run by proprietary organizations; 52 percent of homes with 200 or more beds were run by nonprofit organizations and 28 percent by state, local, or federal government.[5] Eighty-one percent of all homes now have proprietary ownership, and this is the major type of ownership for all homes up to 299 beds. Nonprofit groups run 43 percent of homes with over 300 beds; government agencies, which run only 4 percent of nursing homes overall, operate 57 percent of those with 500 beds or more (44 of 77).

Tables 6-4 and 6-5 show trends over time in bed size, ownership, and staffing levels for homes with 25 or more beds. The percentage owned by government, proprietary, and nonprofit agencies has remained remarkably stable. The average number of full-time equivalent employees increased overall by 13 percent between 1969 and 1980, but the increase was less in the proprietary than in other sectors. Since 1973, nonprofit nursing homes have had a markedly higher ratio of employees per 100 beds than proprietary homes.

Characteristics of Residents

According to the 1977 NNHS, 86 percent of the total nursing home population was aged 65 and over; of the elderly nursing home residents, 40 percent were aged 85 and over (Table 6-6). Nearly 22 percent of the total population of the United States aged 85 and over in 1977 were living in nursing homes (see Table 6-7).[16]

Table 6-8 shows the distribution of nursing home residents by age, sex, race, marital status, and primary source of payment. In addition to

Table 6-3. Beds per 1,000 population aged 65 and over in nursing and related care homes, with 25 or more beds, by state, selected years, 1969-1980.

State	1969	1973	1976	1980
United States	43.4	56.8	56.3	57.2
Alabama	34.8	41.2	49.6	46.9
Alaska	24.6	73.0	82.0	85.8
Arizona	33.3	30.6	24.6	29.1
Arkansas	53.1	68.8	69.5	61.6
California	51.8	64.3	55.7	59.7
Colorado	63.4	80.3	81.6	70.0
Connecticut	54.0	70.4	65.9	53.6
Delaware	26.2	43.1	40.8	41.3
District of Columbia	27.3	39.5	36.7	40.3
Florida	26.1	28.7	23.3	21.3
Georgia	37.5	63.3	64.9	57.4
Hawaii	28.5	39.1	29.4	24.1
Idaho	45.0	52.4	52.6	45.2
Illinois	47.5	67.8	71.6	69.7
Indiana	48.4	63.0	65.9	75.1
Iowa	71.1	88.2	86.1	87.7
Kansas	56.1	74.3	75.0	81.9
Kentucky	34.2	47.9	53.3	62.9
Louisiana	39.2	50.8	53.4	53.6
Maine	30.9	57.3	54.9	63.5
Maryland	46.0	51.6	53.0	51.5
Massachusetts	55.0	75.1	69.5	67.7
Michigan	42.7	58.0	64.7	67.5
Minnesota	71.8	93.6	85.4	86.3
Mississippi	17.2	30.9	32.5	41.9
Missouri	43.8	54.7	53.3	65.7
Montana	37.5	56.3	61.4	63.6
Nebraska	61.0	85.3	93.4	89.8
Nevada	22.1	29.3	28.1	27.8
New Hampshire	37.8	58.4	61.9	62.3
New Jersey	32.6	40.7	39.5	41.2
New Mexico	30.3	36.0	26.5	22.8
New York	32.4	40.7	47.3	46.9
North Carolina	33.3	39.1	40.8	47.1
North Dakota	80.2	88.2	85.5	79.4
Ohio	42.6	55.6	55.7	63.3
Oklahoma	78.5	89.8	76.2	71.8
Oregon	57.9	68.3	59.0	56.4
Pennsylvania	37.2	47.2	41.9	49.3
Rhode Island	38.1	48.6	58.3	66.1
South Carolina	27.4	35.6	34.8	39.3
South Dakota	66.2	87.3	93.6	93.2
Tennessee	26.0	33.0	42.9	41.3
Texas	53.4	72.7	77.9	73.8
Utah	36.2	40.4	39.0	45.7
Vermont	33.9	61.9	65.6	63.1
Virginia	24.7	36.3	54.1	49.2
Washington	54.7	87.6	78.4	85.8
West Virginia	10.8	17.7	22.6	24.9
Wisconsin	55.5	100.1	89.0	87.4
Wyoming	36.2	53.8	51.6	47.5

Source: National Center for Health Statistics, G. W. Strahan: Trends in in nursing and related care homes and hospitals, United States, selected years 1969-80. Vital and Health Statistics, Series 14, No. 30, DHHS Pub. No. (PHS)84-1825. Washington, D.C., U.S. Government Printing Office, March 1984.

Table 6-4. Number and percentage distribution of nursing and related care homes with 25 or more beds, by bed size and type of ownership, selected years, 1969-1980.

	1969	1973	1976	1980
	Number			
All homes	11,465	14,089	14,133	14,567
Bed size				
25 - 49	4,625	4,382	3,666	3,030
50 - 74	2,904	3,452	3,485	3,332
75 - 99	1,627	2,220	2,297	2,375
100 - 199	1,933	3,309	3,863	4,737
200 - 299	254	504	577	766
300 - 499	93	163	181	250
500 or more	29	59	64	77
Type of ownership				
Government	691	963	1,006	883
Federal	15	24	24	14
State & local	676	939	982	869
Proprietary	8,296	10,236	10,300	10,689
Nonprofit	2,478	2,890	2,827	2,995
	Percentage			
All homes	100.0	100.0	100.0	100.0
Bed size				
25 - 49	38.7	29.6	25.9	20.8
50 - 74	27.0	26.0	24.7	22.9
75 - 99	14.2	15.8	16.3	16.3
100 - 199	16.9	23.5	27.3	32.5
200 - 299	2.2	3.6	4.1	5.3
300 - 499	0.8	1.2	1.3	1.7
500 or more	0.3	0.4	0.5	0.5
Type of ownership				
Government	6.0	6.8	7.1	6.1
Federal	0.1	0.2	0.2	0.1
State & local	5.9	6.7	6.9	6.0
Proprietary	72.4	72.7	72.9	73.4
Nonprofit	21.6	20.5	20.0	20.5

Source: National Center for Health Statistics, G.W. Strahan: Trends in nursing and related care homes and hospitals, United States selected years 1969-1980. Vital and Health Statistics, Series 14, No. 30. Series 14 - No. 30. DHHS Pub. No. (PHS)84-1825. Washington, D.C., U.S. Government Printing Office, March 1984.

advanced age, the major characteristics of those admitted to nursing homes are that they are female (71 percent), widowed or never married (81 percent), and white (92 percent). In 1977 only 107 per 1,000 black persons aged 85 and over were resident in nursing homes, compared with 229 per 1,000 white individuals in this age group.[17]

Table 6-5. Full-time equivalent employees per 100 beds in nursing and related care homes with 25 or more beds, by bed size and type of ownership, selected years, 1969-1980.

Bed size and type of ownership	1980*	1976	1973	1969
FTE employees	62.9	57.1	57.2	55.0
Bed size				
25-49 beds	58.0	55.4	53.9	53.1
50-74 beds	61.7	56.1	56.5	55.9
75-99 beds	64.1	57.2	59.1	57.0
100-199 beds	62.3	56.7	58.4	55.6
200-299 beds	63.0	57.9	58.8	54.3
300-499 beds	61.7	57.2	57.9	51.1
500 or more beds	81.4	68.0	48.4	49.6
Type of ownership				
Government	82.2	72.4	63.6	51.9
Federal	49.9	37.1	24.2	26.1
State and local	82.8	73.5	65.2	52.9
Proprietary	59.4	53.3	55.8	55.4
Nonprofit	66.1	62.1	58.6	55.2

*Data were estimated for homes that did not provide counts of their employees.

Source: National Center for Health Statistics, G.W. Strahan: Trends in nursing and related care homes and hospitals, United States, selected years 1969-1980. Vital and Health Statistics, Series 14, No. 30, DHHS Pub. No. (PHS)84-1825. Washington, D.C., U.S. Government Printing Office, March 1984.

Table 6-6. Number and percentage distribution of nursing home residents by age, 1977.

	Number	Percentage	
Total residents	1,303,100	100	Percentage
Age 65 & over	1,126,000	86	100
65-74	211,400	16	19
75-84	464,700	35	41
85-94	405,000	31	36
95 & over	44,900	3	4

Source: National Center for Health Statistics: The National Nursing Home Survey, Summary for the United States, 1977. Vital and Health Statistics, Series 13, No. 43, DHEW Pub. No. (PHS)79-1794. Washington, D.C., U.S. Government Printing Office, July 1979.

Table 6-7.   Comparison of nursing home resident population and the general population, by age, 1977.

| | | Nursing home residents | |
Age	Total population	Number	Percentage of general population
65 & over	23,494,000	1,126,000	4.8
65 - 74	14,584,000	211,400	1.4
75 - 84	6,831,000	464,700	6.8
85 & over	2,079,000	449,900	21.6

Source: National Center for Health Statistics: The National Nursing Home Survey, Summary for the United States, 1977. Vital and Health Statistics, Series 13, No. 43, DHEW Pub. No. (PHS)79-1794.   Washington, D.C., U.S. Government Printing Office, July 1979.

The primary source of payment was Medicaid for 48 percent and self-pay for 38 percent of the total nursing home population. In contrast, Medicaid was the primary source of payment for 73 percent of blacks, with only 13 percent self-pay.

Table 6-9 shows the distribution of nursing home residents by index of dependency in ADL's, for selected characteristics. Ten percent of all nursing home residents were classified as "independent." Dependency levels increase with age for both the nursing home and the noninstitutionalized populations, but there is a higher percentage of total dependency among the nursing home population than for those living in the community in comparable age groups.[17,19] Higher dependency levels were shown for women compared with men. Among those receiving "skilled nursing," 42 percent of Medicare patients were totally dependent compared with 33 percent of Medicaid patients. The lowest dependency levels were found for private pay and "intermediate care" Medicaid patients. It is notable that whereas community studies have shown blacks to have higher levels of functional disability than whites, dependency levels of blacks and whites were comparable in the nursing home population. In terms of marital status, the highest dependency levels were among the married, who constitute only 12 percent of the total nursing home population.

The 1977 NNHS also demonstrated that length of stay increases with age, from a mean of 883 days for those aged 65 to 74 to 1,042 days for those aged 85 and over.[16]

Medicare and Medicaid Utilization

Over 40 percent of all nursing and related care homes included in the NMFI are not certified for Medicare or Medicaid. Data from the 1981

Table 6-8. Number of nursing home residents and percentage distribution by primary source of payment and by sex, age, marital status and race, 1977.

	All sources	Primary source of payment				
					Medicaid	
		Self pay	Medicare	SNF	ICF	All other
			Number			
All residents	1,303,100	500,900	26,200	260,700	362,600	152,600
Sex						
Male	375,300	145,800	7,900	63,400	98,100	60,100
Female	927,800	355,200	18,300	197,300	264,500	92,600
Age						
Under 65 years	177,100	46,500	1,300	32,800	59,700	36,700
65 - 74	211,400	70,800	6,200	40,000	67,900	26,300
75 - 84	464,700	201,900	11,900	88,200	115,800	46,900
85 & over	449,900	181,700	6,800	99,600	119,100	42,700
Marital status						
Married	155,400	77,200	4,400	23,100	30,100	20,500
Widowed	810,700	325,500	18,600	171,300	219,000	76,300
Divorced or septd.	87,500	24,200		19,200	27,500	15,800
Never married	249,500	74,100	2,400	47,000	86,000	39,900
Race						
White	1,200,900	486,600	24,200	233,500	320,000	136,500
Black	81,400	10,700	1,400	21,000	38,200	10,100
Hispanic or other	20,800	3,600		6,200	4,400	6,000

Percentage

	100.0	38.4	2.0	20.0	27.8	11.7
All residents	100.0	38.4	2.0	20.0	27.8	11.7
Sex						
Male	100.0	38.8	2.1	16.9	26.1	16.0
Female	100.0	38.3	2.0	21.3	28.5	10.0
Age						
Under 65 years	100.0	26.2	0.8	18.5	33.7	20.8
65 - 74	100.0	33.5	3.0	18.9	32.1	12.5
75 - 84	100.0	43.4	2.6	19.0	24.9	10.0
85 & over	100.0	40.4	1.5	22.1	26.5	9.5
Marital status						
Married	100.0	49.7	2.8	14.9	19.4	13.3
Widowed	100.0	40.1	2.3	21.1	27.0	9.4
Divorced or septd.	100.0	27.6		22.0	31.4	18.1
Never married	100.0	29.7	1.8	18.8	34.5	16.0
Race						
White	100.0	40.5	2.0	19.4	26.7	11.4
Black	100.0	13.1	1.8	25.8	46.9	12.4
Hispanic or other	100.0	17.5		29.7	21.0	29.2

Source: National Center for Health Statistics: Hing E., Characteristics of nursing home residents, health status and care received. The National Nursing Home Survey, 1977. Vital and Health Statistics: Series 13, No. 51, DHHS Publication No. (PHS)81-1712. Washington, D.C., U.S. Government Printing Office, April 1981.

Table 6-9. Number and percentage distribution of nursing home residents by index of dependency in activities of daily living, by selected resident characteristics, 1977.

Index of dependency in activities of daily living *

Selected resident characteristic	Total	Independent	Dependent in one activity	Dependent in bathing and one other activity	Dependent in bathing, dressing, and one other activity	Dependent in bathing, dressing, using toilet and one other activity	Dependent in bathing, dressing, using toilet, mobility, and one other activity	Dependent in all six activities
				Percentage distribution				
Total	100.0	9.6	12.4	12.2	8.5	9.6	15.6	23.3
Sex								
Male	100.0	13.5	15.1	13.8	7.3	7.4	14.0	19.1
Female	100.0	7.9	11.3	11.6	8.9	10.5	16.3	24.9
Age								
Under 65	100.0	23.4	15.6	12.9	7.2	6.7	12.8	15.7
65 & over	100.0	7.4	11.9	12.1	8.7	10.1	16.1	24.5
65–74	100.0	14.0	16.5	13.4	6.7	9.9	15.2	17.6
75–84	100.0	7.2	12.3	11.7	9.6	10.5	15.3	24.3
85 & over	100.0	4.4	9.2	11.9	8.6	9.7	17.3	27.9

Race or ethnicity

White (not Hispanic)**	100.0	9.5	12.6	12.1	8.5	9.6	15.4	23.3
Black (not Hispanic)	100.0	9.3	9.0	12.8	8.7	9.8	19.1	22.9
Hispanic and other	100.0	13.3	11.5	15.0	6.2	6.3	17.0	20.7

Marital status

Married	100.0	7.8	8.6	7.4	6.7	9.5	19.4	30.8
Widowed **	100.0	6.4	11.3	12.0	9.3	10.2	16.7	24.8
Divorced or septd.	100.0	21.0	16.2	14.2	7.2	7.2	13.0	15.1
Never married	100.0	16.8	16.9	15.2	7.3	8.6	10.7	16.6

Primary payment source

Own / family income	100.0	10.1	13.2	11.9	8.0	9.7	16.0	21.6
Medicare	100.0	–	–	–	5.7	19.5	17.7	41.5
Medicaid:	100.0							
Skilled	100.0	3.2	5.7	9.0	7.8	10.4	20.1	32.9
Intermediate	100.0	9.6	16.1	16.0	10.3	8.6	13.5	18.5

* Unknowns were considered independent for the purpose of this index.

** Includes a small number of unknowns

Source: National Center for Health Statistics. National Nursing Home Survey, Summary for the United States, 1977. Vital and Health Statistics, Series 13, No.43, DHEW Publication No. (PHS)79-1794. Washington, D.C., U.S. Government Printing Office, July 1979.

MMACS showed that 13,323 homes were certified for Medicare and/or Medicaid compared with 23,065 included in the 1980 NMFI. The majority of the additional 10,000 homes consists of those that accept only private patients and have not sought Medicare and/or Medicaid reimbursements. There are, in addition, homes that may have failed to meet certification standards and others that receive payments for residents from the Supplemental Security Income program (see below).

MMACS data for 1981 showed only 6 percent of all Medicare and/or Medicaid certified facilities (761 of 13,326) to be hospital-based nursing home units, 83 percent being SNF's. In view of changes in the Medicare system, with the incentive for hospitals to discharge patients more rapidly from acute care hospitals under the diagnosis-related group (DRG) system, hospital-based nursing homes may become a progressively more important sector of the long-term care market, particularly where there is a surplus of hospital beds.

As with the NMFI's, data from the 1981 MMACS on nursing homes certified for Medicare and Medicaid also show wide variation by state in the number of beds per 1,000 total population, population aged 65 and over and, most important, the population aged 85 and over—the sector with the greatest utilization of services. The latter ratio varies from less than 150 in Arizona and the District of Columbia to 895 in Wisconsin (see Table 6-10).

Variations across the country in administration of the Medicare and Medicaid programs, and difficulties associated with implementing the "level of care" concept, which distinguishes between the need for "skilled nursing" and "intermediate care," have led to inconsistent patterns of utilization and reimbursement for nursing home care.

Regardless of the percentage of the population aged 65 and over or the size of the Medicaid-eligible population, the number and percentage of beds certified for Medicare and/or Medicaid and the relative proportions of SNF's and ICF's vary greatly by state (see Tables 6-11 and 6-12). MMACS data for 1981 show that whereas less than 10 percent of beds were certified for both Medicare and Medicaid in some states, such as Texas, Utah, and Arkansas, in other states, such as New York, Alabama, and Nevada, over 90 percent were dually certified, with many nursing homes adapting bed usage between "skilled nursing" and "intermediate care."

Table 6-12 shows the variation by state in the number of Medicare-reimbursed SNF days per 1,000 persons aged 65 and over in 1979. The range was from a high of 691 days in Hawaii to a low of 58 in Mississippi, with a mean of 326 nationally. Under Medicare reimbursement regulations there can be retroactive denial of eligibility and payments for patients already admitted to nursing homes, and major differences have been documented between fiscal intermediaries in the interpretation of the rules governing the Medicare benefit. Therefore, many nursing homes

Table 6-10. Total beds in certified facilities, beds per 1,000 population, beds per 1,000 population aged 65 and over and beds per 1,000 population aged 85 and over, by state, 1981.

State	Total beds	Beds per 1000 population	Beds per 1,000 population aged 65 & over	Beds per 1,000 population aged 85 & over
United States	1,362,223	5.9	53.4	558.2
Alabama	20,742	5.3	47.5	546.4
Alaska	644	1.6	54.6	825.6
Arizona	3,217	1.2	10.4	147.3
Arkansas	19,574	8.5	63.8	698.6
California	114,468	4.7	47.7	487.1
Colorado	18,936	6.4	75.7	726.2
Connecticut	24,783	7.9	66.8	638.5
Delaware	2,789	4.7	45.9	491.0
District of Columbia	1,166	1.8	16.6	144.7
Florida	34,705	3.4	21.3	270.7
Georgia	30,649	5.5	59.9	715.0
Hawaii	2,516	2.6	32.4	414.4
Idaho	4,769	4.9	48.8	532.4
Illinois	90,107	7.9	71.7	725.5
Indiana	41,604	7.6	70.5	731.6
Iowa	34,118	11.8	87.1	721.5
Kansas	25,694	10.8	83.6	726.3
Kentucky	20,304	5.5	49.8	540.7
Louisiana	24,648	5.7	63.9	659.4
Maine	9,140	8.1	63.2	592.9
Maryland	20,909	4.9	53.5	583.6
Massachusetts	45,005	7.8	62.2	553.4
Michigan	46,275	5.0	49.4	524.9
Minnesota	46,335	11.3	95.0	811.8
Mississippi	12,294	4.9	43.3	447.7
Missouri	26,243	5.3	40.7	398.0
Montana	6,334	8.0	72.2	681.0
Nebraska	17,425	11.0	84.1	694.7
Nevada	2,269	2.7	32.6	534.4
New Hampshire	6,740	7.2	63.7	642.5
New Jersey	32,232	4.3	37.2	404.7
New Mexico	3,565	2.7	30.1	352.4
New York	94,124	5.3	44.0	424.3
North Carolina	21,722	3.6	35.8	440.8
North Dakota	6,570	10.0	79.3	746.0
Ohio	70,799	6.6	59.8	610.7
Oklahoma	28,330	9.1	77.3	794.2
Oregon	14,868	5.6	48.1	488.7
Pennsylvania	68,969	5.8	44.7	488.0
Rhode Island	8,545	9.0	67.5	622.0
South Carolina	10,880	3.4	37.8	489.0
South Dakota	7,880	11.5	84.9	705.6
Tennessee	24,540	5.3	47.9	552.0
Texas	100,059	6.8	74.4	846.0
Utah	5,214	3.4	46.5	538.0
Vermont	2,982	5.8	50.3	466.7
Virginia	20,428	3.8	40.6	490.8
Washington	24,872	5.9	56.7	561.0
West Virginia	5,721	2.9	24.2	275.1
Wisconsin	53,617	11.3	92.7	895.0
Wyoming	1,904	3.9	49.2	506.6

Source: Health Care Financing Administration, Office of Research and Demonstrations. Unpublished data based on the Medicare and Medicaid Automated Certification System, 1981.

Table 6-11. Total beds in certified facilities, percentage certified for Medicare and Medicaid, and percentage certified for Medicaid only, by state, 1981.

	All certified beds	Percentage Medicare/ Medicaid	Percentage Medicaid only
United States	1,362,223	47	53
Alabama	20,742	94	9
Alaska	644	50	50
Arizona	3,217	100	0
Arkansas	19,574	3	96
California	114,468	80	20
Colorado	18,936	39	61
Connecticut	24,783	87	12
Delaware	2,789	55	46
District of Columbia	1,166	47	53
Florida	34,705	71	29
Georgia	30,649	27	74
Hawaii	2,516	78	23
Idaho	4,769	70	30
Illinois	90,107	36	64
Indiana	41,604	44	56
Iowa	34,118	7	94
Kansas	25,694	10	90
Kentucky	20,304	50	49
Louisiana	24,648	7	92
Maine	9,140	14	87
Maryland	20,909	63	37
Massachusetts	45,005	32	69
Michigan	46,275	76	25
Minnesota	46,335	23	77
Mississippi	12,294	9	91
Missouri	26,243	26	74
Montana	6,334	71	29
Nebraska	17,425	11	89
Nevada	2,269	92	8
New Hampshire	6,740	34	66
New Jersey	32,232	54	46
New Mexico	3,565	17	84
New York	94,124	93	7
North Carolina	21,722	70	30
North Dakota	6,570	73	27
Ohio	70,799	60	40
Oklahoma	28,330	3	97
Oregon	14,868	34	66
Pennsylvania	68,969	72	27
Rhode Island	8,545	78	22
South Carolina	10,880	81	19
South Dakota	7,880	7	94
Tennessee	24,540	32	68
Texas	100,059	6	94
Utah	5,214	41	58
Vermont	2,982	56	43
Virginia	20,428	42	58
Washington	24,872	40	60
West Virginia	5,721	53	47
Wisconsin	53,617	21	79
Wyoming	1,904	9	91

Source: Health Care Financing Administration: Office of Research and Demonstrations. Unpublished data based on the Medicare and Medicaid Automated Certification System, 1981.

Table 6-12. Medicare certified skilled nursing facility beds and Medicare reimbursed days per 1,000 persons aged 65 and over, by state, 1979

	Total Medicare SNF beds	Percentage SNF beds certified for Medicare	Medicare SNF days/1000 aged 65 & over	Rank
United States	419,835	67.1	326.2	-
Hawaii	2,089	100	691	1
Ohio	24,192	78.6	561	2
Kentucky	4,386	100	552.6	3
North Dakota	3,929	100	548	4
Nevada	1,702	100	533.5	5
New Hampshire	835	100	512.7	6
Michigan	22,193	91.6	499.1	7
Pennsylvania	29,917	74	475.8	8
Illinois	9,327	30	465	9
North Carolina	7,927	94.8	463.8	10
Montana	2,903	85.3	459.7	11
Oregon	3,632	91.7	425.9	12
Utah	1,841	68.7	419.9	13
Alabama	12,274	99.3	419.8	14
Rhode Island	1,801	98.4	414	15
South Carolina	6,068	100	401.6	16
Indiana	5,957	85.7	381.4	17
Florida	19,416	68.7	381.4	18
California	87,821	86	378	19
Washington	10,167	39.7	343.2	20
Maryland	6,930	100	340.2	21
New Jersey	13,950	61.9	335.6	22
Delaware	857	97.8	333.5	23
Tennessee	2,640	100	320	24
Missouri	3,897	53.3	301.6	25
Nebraska	1,380	50.9	278.2	26
Vermont	698	90.4	275.9	27
Idaho	3,014	68.7	268.3	28
Maine	609	100	264.1	29
New York	67,079	99.7	262.9	30
Virginia	1,765	100	243.4	31
District of Columbia	491	100	234.1	32
Arizona	784	100	230.5	33
Iowa	819	97.7	224.1	34
West Virginia	2,703	100	219.7	35
Massachusetts	6,650	45.9	198.5	36
Wisconsin	5,732	21.1	187.4	37
Connecticut	16,743	92	181.3	38
Colorado	5,918	50.7	172	39
Georgia	5,126	28.6	160.3	40
South Dakota	393	12.6	156	41
Wyoming	273	12.1	149.5	42
Minnesota	5,241	17.6	148.5	43
Kansas	1,702	42.4	144.7	44
Louisiana	1,838	100	141	45
Oklahoma	353	100	118.4	46
Alaska	207	62.4	110.4	47
Texas	2,402	16.1	95.3	48
New Mexico	223	100	94.1	49
Arkansas	314	3.6	58.5	50
Mississippi	546	5.4	57.9	51

Source: Health Care Financing Administration: Medicare and Medicaid Automated Certification System, and Project to Analyze Existing Long-Term Care Data, Volume 1V: Financing Long-Term Care. The Urban Institute, Washington D.C. 1983.

do not choose to participate in the Medicare program, and it has been described as the "underused benefit."[20,21]

Medicaid programs make coverage decisions in advance of treatment, award longer periods of coverage than Medicare for similar cases, and do not require detailed documentation of the patients' condition or of service delivery. Consequently, many facilities accept the higher Medicaid SNF payment and do not apply for Medicare certification.[21]

Medicaid utilization also varies considerably by state, particularly in relationship to SNF and ICF care. Table 6-13 demonstrates that in 1983 the percentage of the total Medicaid population receiving SNF care ranged from a high of 10 percent in North Dakota, followed by Connecticut and Minnesota with over 8 percent, to 0 percent in Maryland, Oklahoma, and West Virginia. The percentage of Medicaid recipients in ICF's ranged from 0.6 percent in California to 17.5 percent in North Dakota. The national mean for the total percentage of Medicaid-reimbursed nursing home recipients, in both SNF's and ICF's, is 7 percent, ranging from 5 percent or less in California, Michigan, and a number of smaller states to more than 18 percent in North Dakota and South Dakota.

Expenditures

Expenditures for nursing home care increased nearly 300 percent between 1965 and 1971 and, as shown in Table 6-14, there was a further 300-percent increase between 1971 and 1979. While private payments accounted for 66 percent of nursing home expenditures in 1965, by 1979 only 44 percent were private payments, because the proportion of public expenditures increased. Since then this trend has been reversed, and in 1983 public expenditures had declined to 48 percent as private expenditures rose to 52 percent of total payments.

Although public financing of nursing home care has increased, Medicare funded only 1.8 percent of total expenditures for nursing home care in 1983. The proportion of the Medicare budget financing the nursing home benefit declined progressively, from 5 percent in 1967 to 2 percent in 1975 and to less than 1 percent in 1981.[22]

State Medicaid programs are the largest purchasers of nursing home care in the country, providing 49 percent of all nursing home payments in 1979, but dropping to 43 percent in 1983. The $12.4 billion in Medicaid expenditures in 1983 represented 88 percent of all public expenditures for nursing home care (see Table 6-14). It is estimated that 60 percent of total Medicaid expenditures for recipients aged 65 and over in 1983 were for nursing home care. If the costs of medical services provided to nursing home residents were included, the proportions would be even higher.[23]

As shown in Table 6-15, 44 percent of total Medicaid budgets in 1983 were expenditures for nursing home care, with a range from 29 percent

Table 6-13. Percentage of all Medicaid recipients in skilled and intermediate care facilities, by state, 1983.

	Skilled	Intermediate	Total
United States	2.7	4.4	7.1
Alabama	1.2	5.9	7.1
Alaska	1.3	3.3	4.6
Arizona			
Arkansas	3.2	9.4	12.6
California	3.5	0.6	4.1
Colorado	3.4	8.0	11.4
Connecticut	8.3	2.4	10.7
Delaware	0.2	4.8	5.0
District of Columbia	0.2	2.5	2.7
Florida	2.4	5.0	7.4
Georgia	3.7	5.0	8.7
Hawaii	2.6	2.9	5.5
Idaho	4.1	7.8	11.9
Illinois	2.1	5.3	7.4
Indiana	3.7	11.5	15.2
Iowa	0.2	11.4	11.6
Kansas	0.6	11.7	12.3
Kentucky	1.6	4.7	6.3
Louisiana	0.3	10.2	10.5
Maine	0.7	8.0	8.7
Maryland	0.0	5.5	5.5
Massachusetts	5.1	5.6	10.7
Michigan	1.6	3.5	5.1
Minnesota	8.4	8.1	16.5
Mississippi	2.4	3.6	6.0
Missouri	0.7	7.7	8.4
Montana	0.5	10.9	11.4
Nebraska	1.3	11.7	13.0
Nevada	1.7	9.1	10.8
New Hampshire	0.5	13.4	13.9
New Jersey	0.8	4.9	5.3
New Mexico	0.3	4.9	5.2
New York	3.7	2.4	6.1
North Carolina	4.0	4.7	8.7
North Dakota	10.1	8.9	19.0
Ohio	3.5	3.7	7.2
Oklahoma	0.0	10.4	10.4
Oregon	0.7	8.6	9.3
Pennsylvania	3.9	4.3	8.2
Rhode Island	1.3	8.3	9.6
South Carolina	2.2	4.8	7.0
South Dakota	1.3	17.5	18.8
Tennessee	1.4	8.1	9.5
Texas	1.0	12.6	13.6
Utah	0.9	8.1	9.0
Vermont	0.3	6.2	6.5
Virginia	0.6	7.3	7.9
Washington	7.8	2.9	10.7
West Virginia	0.0	5.2	5.2
Wisconsin	6.8	5.6	12.4
Wyoming	1.9	9.3	11.2

Source: Health Care Financing Administration, Annual Statistical Report on Medical Care Recipients, Payments and Services. HCFA 2082, 1983. Office of Financial and Actuarial Analysis, Division of Medical Cost Estimates, Medical Statistics Branch.

Table 6-14. Calendar year estimates of expenditures for nursing home care, in millions of dollars, by source of payment and as a percentage of total payments, selected years, 1965-1983.

	1965		1968	
	Amount	Percentage	Amount	Percentage
Total:	2,072	100.0	3,380	100.0
Public payments:	712	34.4	1,780	52.7
Medicaid	-	-	1,137	33.6
Medicare	-	-	396	11.7
Veterans Administration	6	0.3	37	1.1
Other	706	34.1	210	6.2
Private payments:	1,360	65.6	1,600	47.3
Direct	1,337	64.5	1,569	46.4
Insurance	2	0.1	8	0.2
Other	21	1.0	24	0.7

	1971		1976	
	Amount	Percentage	Amount	Percentage
Total:	5,635	100.0	11,319	100.0
Public payments:	2,824	50.1	6,257	55.3
Medicaid	1,926	34.2	5,352	47.3
Medicare	182	3.2	327	2.9
Veterans Administration	82	1.5	208	1.8
Other	633	11.2	371	3.2
Private payments:	2,811	49.9	5,061	44.7
Direct	2,750	48.8	4,903	43.3
Insurance	22	0.4	88	0.8
Other	39	0.7	70	0.6

	1979		1983	
	Amount	Percentage	Amount	Percentage
Total:	17,406	100.0	28,838	100.0
Public payments:	9,727	55.9	13,960	48.4
Medicaid	8,463	48.6	12,354	42.8
Medicare	368	2.1	529	1.8
Veterans Administration	312	1.8	542	1.9
Other	584	3.4	535	1.9
Private payments:	7,679	44.1	14,878	51.6
Direct	7,433	42.7	14,403	49.9
Insurance	140	0.8	269	0.9
Other	106	0.6	206	0.7

Source: Health Care Financing Administration, Office of Financial and Actuarial Analysis, Division of Medical Cost Estimates. Published and unpublished data.

in the District of Columbia to over 60 percent in Connecticut, Minnesota, Idaho, and New Hampshire. A comparison of Table 6-13 with Table 6-15 reveals the high proportion of the Medicaid population in nursing homes. On average, 7 percent of eligible individuals in 1983 received 44 percent of Medicaid expenditures.

Table 6-15. Total Medicaid expenditures, by state, and percentage of total expenditures for skilled and intermediate care, 1983.

	Total payments (thousands of dollars)	Percentage skilled	Percentage intermediate	Percentage skilled and intermediate
United States	32,350,546	14.3	29.2	43.5
Alabama	368,732	2.6	43.0	45.6
Alaska	51,247	5.2	40.7	45.9
Arizona				
Arkansas	313,207	9.9	40.7	50.7
California	3,557,151	18.9	13.6	32.4
Colorado	255,304	10.9	43.2	54.1
Connecticut	459,413	44.8	15.6	60.4
Delaware	62,084	0.5	47.4	47.9
District of Columbia	196,543	1.5	27.4	28.9
Florida	681,263	8.3	33.1	41.4
Georgia	601,435	11.2	25.2	36.4
Hawaii	141,689	16.9	29.7	46.6
Idaho	67,257	11.9	49.5	61.5
Illinois	1,347,004	7.7	34.1	41.8
Indiana	596,027	10.6	39.2	49.8
Iowa	312,041	0.7	49.4	50.1
Kansas	254,478	0.7	47.5	48.2
Kentucky	410,998	7.8	31.9	39.6
Louisiana	674,703	0.9	53.0	53.9
Maine	205,071	1.4	50.1	51.5
Maryland	446,636	0.0	37.6	37.6
Massachusetts	1,338,237	16.2	29.2	45.4
Michigan	1,421,703	6.7	29.2	35.9
Minnesota	868,114	30.5	34.9	65.5
Mississippi	299,390	15.5	27.7	43.3
Missouri	468,458	1.3	49.6	50.8
Montana	86,169	1.5	49.1	50.6
Nebraska	145,962	5.0	47.8	52.8
Nevada	73,706	2.5	38.1	40.7
New Hampshire	93,100	1.0	63.9	64.9
New Jersey	981,530	2.6	40.5	43.1
New Mexico	101,780	1.6	34.7	36.3
New York	6,259,549	23.3	16.7	40.0
North Carolina	566,992	17.0	31.3	48.2
North Dakota	83,319	32.2	24.9	57.2
Ohio	1,474,339	15.1	21.9	37.1
Oklahoma	388,659	0.1	43.7	43.8
Oregon	236,231	1.3	46.3	47.6
Pennsylvania	1,718,810	18.7	36.5	55.3
Rhode Island	221,733	1.4	51.9	53.3
South Carolina	278,833	12.6	39.1	51.7
South Dakota	77,792	2.0	54.3	56.3
Tennessee	508,566	3.2	44.5	47.7
Texas	1,316,684	2.6	50.7	53.2
Utah	114,518	2.2	45.7	48.0
Vermont	84,272	0.9	47.7	48.7
Virginia	488,158	2.4	51.1	53.4
Washington	427,141	31.5	22.6	54.2
West Virginia	140,626	0.0	37.7	37.7
Wisconsin	901,103	29.2	27.1	56.2
Wyoming	24,445	6.6	45.3	52.0

Source: Health Care Financing Administration: Annual Statistical Report on Medical Care Recipients, Payments and Services. HCFA 2082, 1983. Office of Financial and Actuarial Analysis, Division of Medical Cost Estimates, Medical Statistics Branch.

In some states, notably California, a high proportion of Medicaid recipients potentially eligible for ICF's, who are in need of personal rather than medical care, have care purchased for them in board and care homes financed through federal support payments made to the individuals under the Supplemental Security Income program (see Chapters 3 and 9). These payments are supplemented by the state at a net cost that is less than if the same care were purchased by the state in a Medicaid-certified ICF.[24] As a result, California has the lowest proportion of total Medicaid expenditures for ICF in the United States (see Table 6-15).

There is additional federal funding of nursing home care through Veterans Administration programs (see Chapter 10).

Future Projections

Table 6-16 shows the number of nursing home residents, by age, in 1977 and the potential nursing home population in the years 2000, 2020, and 2050 based on 1977 utilization rates and recent projections of the future population of the United States. The estimates for the future are substantially higher than those published before the 1980 population census,[23] which documented the higher than previously anticipated growth in the numbers of very elderly in the population.

At 1977 utilization rates, it is predicted that 85 percent of the present stock of nursing home beds will be occupied by those aged 85 and over in the year 2000.

Table 6-16. Distribution of nursing home residents by age in 1977, and projections of the number in selected years, based on 1977 utilization rates.

| | | Nursing home residents | | |
| | Actual numbers | | Projections | |
Age group	1977	2000	2020	2050
Total	1,270,300	2,346,430	3,220,043	5,608,114
45-54	43,500	70,530	68,742	70,285
55-64	100,800	116,460	202,360	182,902
65-74	211,400	256,320	432,898	436,653
75-84	464,700	840,090	987,945	1,450,137
85 & over	449,900	1,063,030	1,528,098	3,460,137

Source: Derived from: National Center for Health Statistics: National Nursing Home Survey, 1977, and U.S. Bureau of the Census, Projections of the Population of the United States: 1983 to 2080. Series P-25, No. 952. Washington, D.C., U.S. Government Printing Office, 1984.

Summary

The implementation of nursing home benefits in the Medicare and Medicaid programs in 1966 was a major impetus to growth and expansion in the nursing home industry, but the rate of increase has slowed in recent years.

Restriction of the Medicare benefit to posthospital "skilled nursing" care has limited expenditures to approximately 1 percent of the Medicare budget. The Medicaid program, on the other hand, has become the major source of public financing for long-term care; over 40 percent of total Medicaid expenditures and 60 percent of those paid on behalf of the elderly are for nursing home care, predominantly in "intermediate care facilities." Fifty percent of nursing home expenditures are paid for out of pocket by individuals or their families, a proportion that has been increasing since 1979.

The highest utilization of nursing home care is by very elderly, white women without spouses. In 1977 22 percent of the total U.S. population aged 85 and over resided in nursing homes and constituted 40 percent of all nursing home residents.

There is wide variation by state in the number of nursing home beds per 1,000 persons aged 65 and over and 85 and over. The ratio of nursing home beds to the total elderly population has remained constant since 1973 in spite of major increases in the proportion of the very elderly.

Nationally, 60 percent of nursing home beds are certified for Medicare and/or Medicaid, but there is wide variation by state in the proportion of beds certified for Medicare or Medicaid and in the ratio of "skilled" to "intermediate care" beds.

Projections of the potential future need for nursing home care should be set in the context of declining rates of growth in the number of nursing home beds in recent years, the increasing constraints on federal program reimbursements, and the economic feasibility and social desirability of major increases in the size of the institutionalized elderly population.

REFERENCES

1. Waldman S. A legislative history of nursing home care. In Vogel R. J. & Palmer H. C. (eds): Long Term Care: Perspectives from Research and Demonstrations. Health Care Financing Administration. U.S. Government Printing Office, 1983.
2. Vladeck B. C. Unloving Care: the nursing home tragedy. New York, Basic Books, 1980.
3. Stevens R. American Medicine and the Public Interest. New Haven and London, Yale University Press, 1971.
4. National Center for Health Statistics, Development and maintenance of a national inventory of hospitals and institutions. Vital and Health Statistics,

Series 1, No.3. DHEW, Pub. No. 1000, Public Health Service, Washington, D.C. U.S. Government Printing Office, February 1965.

5. National Center for Health Statistics, Inpatient health facilities as reported from the 1967 MFI survey. Vital and Health Statistics, Series 14, No.4. DHEW Pub. No. (HSM) 72-1065, Public Health Service, Washington, D.C. U.S. Government Printing Office, June 1972.

6. National Center for Health Statistics, Inpatient health facilities as reported from the 1969 MFI survey. Vital and Health Statistics, Series 14, No. 6. DHEW Pub. No. (HSM) 73-1801, Public Health Service, Washington, D.C. U.S. Government Printing Office, December 1972.

7. National Center for Health Statistics, Inpatient health facilities as reported from the 1971 MFI survey. Vital and Health Statistics, Series 14, No.12. DHEW Pub. No. (HRA) 74-1807, Public Health Service, Washington, D.C. U.S. Government Printing Office, March 1974.

8. National Center for Health Statistics, Inpatient health facilities as reported from the 1973 MFI survey. Vital and Health Statistics, Series 14, No.16. DHEW Pub. No. (HRA) 76-1811, Public Health Service, Washington, D.C. U.S. Government Printing Office, May 1976.

9. National Center for Health Statistics, Inpatient health facilities as reported from the 1976 MFI survey. Vital and Health Statistics, Series 14, No. 23. DHEW Pub. No. (PHS) 80-1818, Public Health Service, Washington, D.C. U.S. Government Printing Office, January 1980.

10. National Center for Health Statistics, Strahan G W.: Inpatient health facilities statistics, United States, 1978. Vital and Health Statistics, Series 14, No. 24. DHEW Pub. No. (PHS) 81-1819, Public Health Service, Washington, D.C. U.S. Government Printing Office, March 1981.

11. National Center for Health Statistics, Sirrocco A.: Nursing and related care homes as reported from the 1980 NMFI survey. Vital and Health Statistics, Series 14, No.29. DHHS Pub. No. (PHS) 84-1824, Public Health Service, Washington, D.C. U.S. Government Printing Office, December 1983.

12. National Center for Health Statistics, Strahan G. W.: Trends in nursing and related care homes and hospitals, United States, selected years 1969–1980. Vital and Health Statistics, Series 14, No.30. DHHS Pub. No. (PHS) 84-1824, Public Health Service, Washington, D.C. U.S. Government Printing Office, December 1983.

13. National Center for Health Statistics, Bryant E. Institutions for the aged and chronically ill, United States, April–June 1963. Vital and Health Statistics, Series 12, No. 2. PHS Pub. No. 1000, Public Health Service, Washington, D.C. U.S. Government Printing Office, July 1965.

14. National Center for Health Statistics, Mathis E. Characteristics of residents in nursing and personal care homes, United States, June–August 1969, Vital and Health Statistics. Series 12, No. 19. DHEW Pub. No. (HSM)73-1704, Public Health Service, Washington, D.C. U.S. Government Printing Office, February 1973.

15. National Center for Health Statistics, Sirrocco A., Koch H. Nursing homes in the United States: 1973–74 National Nursing Home Survey. Vital and Health Statistics Series 14, No. 17. DHEW Pub. No. (HRA) 78-1812, Public Health Service, Washington, D.C. U.S. Government Printing Office, October 1977.

16. National Center for Health Statistics, The National Nursing Home Survey: 1977 Summary for the United States. Vital and Health Statistics, Series 13 No. 43, DHEW Pub. No. (PHS)79-1794, Public Health Service, Washington, D.C. U.S. Government Printing Office, July 1979.
17. National Center for Health Statistics. Hing E. Characteristics of nursing home residents, health status and care received. The National Nursing Home Survey, United States, May–Dec 1977. Vital and Health Statistics, Series 13-No. 51. DHHS Pub. No. (PHS) 81-1712, Public Health Service, Washington, D.C. U.S. Government Printing Office, April 1981.
18. National Center for Health Statistics, Sirrocco A. Unpublished data from the 1982 Master Facility Inventory, 1985.
19. Macken C. L. Descriptive profile of the functionally impaired aged living in the community: findings from the 1982 Long-Term Care Survey. Office of Research and Demonstrations, Health Care Financing Administration, draft report, 1985.
20. Smits H. L., Feder J., Scanlon W. Medicare's nursing-home benefit: variations in interpretation. New England Journal of Medicine 307: 855-862, 1982.
21. Feder J., Scanlon W. The underused benefit: Medicare's coverage of nursing home care. Milbank Memorial Fund Quarterly 60, 4, 604–632, 1982.
22. National Center for Health Statistics, Health, United States, 1983. DHHS Pub. No. (PHS)84-1232, Public Health Service, Washington, D.C. U.S. Government Printing Office, December 1983.
23. Fox P. D., Clauser S. B. Trends in nursing home expenditures: implications for aging policy. Health Care Financing Review 2: 2: 65–70, 1980.
24. Feder J., Scanlon W. Fiscal incentives in federal-state financing for long-term care, in Vol IV, Project to Analyze Existing Long-Term Care Data, The Urban Institute, Washington, D.C. 1983.

7

Home Care: The Population and the System

The provision of nursing and other personal and supportive care services in the home has less of a tradition in the United States than in many European countries, but the field of home care has assumed greater importance with the growing need for long-term care services and the search for alternatives to high-cost institutional care, whether provided in the acute hospital or the nursing home.

The terms "home care" and "home health care" encompass a range or combination of services in which the home is usually the site of service delivery and in which there may be significant involvement of family and friends of the recipient in the care-giving process.[1] Home care ranges from nursing and rehabilitation services provided by skilled personnel, to assistance with personal hygiene and home management, to help with shopping or making telephone calls. It may form part of a spectrum of care, complementing adult day care and other service programs. Utilization depends on service availability, eligibility, medical and functional criteria, and other indicators, including the preference of the client and family for the avoidance of institutional care.

A three- or four-part classification for home care has been developed with the following definitions.

> *Intensive*—Involves a large medical component, featuring extensive use of medical personnel in a home setting, into which high-technology apparatus may be introduced. The objective is to complement and shorten the hospital stay.

> *Intermediate*—Largely unspecified, but usually including medical and nursing input combined with some of the maintenance aspects of basic care. The objectives include the prevention or reduction of hospital and nursing home admissions.

> *Basic*—A combination of maintenance and personal care with the purpose of maintaining people in their own homes at effective levels of health and functioning over long periods of time, or permanently,

without recourse to more concentrated care or to permanent institutionalization.[1]

The Home Care Population

In general terms, the home care population may be defined as all noninstitutionalized individuals needing help from at least one other person because of an acute or chronic medical condition and/or functional disability. Care may range from short-term assistance during or after an episode of acute illness or long-term assistance aimed at continuing home maintenance of disabled and/or dependent individuals who would otherwise be at risk of institutionalization.

It has been shown that professional home health care visits are made to individuals of all ages, a high proportion of whom are not limited in activity and consider themselves to be in good or excellent health.[2] The same study, however, showed a more intensive pattern of utilization among the elderly, who were also more likely to be limited in activity than younger users.

The successful maintenance of elderly, disabled individuals at home depends on a complex relationship between age, family structure, disease state and level of functioning, availability of home and community support services, and eligibility for publicly funded services or ability to pay privately for needed care.

Home Care Financing

Federal funding for home care is provided under Medicare, Medicaid, Title XX of the Social Security Act, Title III of the Older Americans Act and through the Veterans Administration, with additional funding available through research and demonstration grants.

Medicare benefits are provided to all eligible enrollees for a restricted range of reimbursable "home health care" services. Medicare eligibility is designed to limit service to conditions that would otherwise require hospitalization. The provisions require that the patient be "homebound" and in need of "skilled" care provided under a physician-written plan.[3]

Medicaid has the potential for making available a wide range of nursing and supportive care services under the federal regulations, but the actual provision, coverage, and eligibility for such services are determined by the individual states. In addition, states have an option to provide "personal care" under Medicaid, distinct from the "health care" provisions.

It was estimated that in 1980 Medicare expenditures accounted for 81 percent of publicly funded home health care, Medicaid for 18 percent, and the Veterans Administration—which has a limited but increasing number of hospital-based home care programs—for 1.0 percent.[4]

Other home care programs may be developed and provided using a combination of federal Title XX and Title III funds together with state revenues and funding from other sources. These are coordinated by State and Area Agencies on Aging that contract with local service providers (see Chapter 9). In fiscal year 1980 it was estimated that 61 percent of public expenditures for nonmedical home care were from the Title XX program, 6 percent from the Older Americans Act, and 33 percent from Medicaid under its "personal care" option.[4]

Private insurance companies are increasingly providing home health benefits, usually following the Medicare benefit structure but with limits on the number of visits and on total reimbursements.[5] In 1977 it was shown that those aged under 65 were more likely to have home health care visits reimbursed by private insurance than the elderly receiving home health care.[2]

Home Care Providers

The vast majority of home care is provided by the "informal network" of family and friends.[6-9] In addition to direct provision of care, there is evidence that where formal providers of home care are needed, a high proportion of expenditures for such care is made by the individual recipients and/or their families.[1,8]

Medicare-reimbursed home health services must be provided by agencies that are certified for participation in the program. In most states the Medicaid population is served by these same agencies, or there is direct provision of care from state agencies. However, there is known to be a large and increasing number of home care agencies that limit their activities to homemaker and home health aide services and serve only private-pay clients. It was estimated in 1983 that there were twice as many such agencies as there were Medicare-certified providers, but no national data are available to document the characteristics of these agencies or their client population.[10]

DATA SOURCES

Sources of information for the tables presented in this chapter are as follows:

The two major information sources on the characteristics of the home care population and the volume and type of services needed are those that yielded prevalence rates for morbidity and functional disability: the Home Care Supplement to the 1979 and 1980 National Health Interview Survey (NHIS)[7,11] and the 1982 National Long-Term Care Survey (NLTCS).[8-9,12-13] The latter has also provided information on sources of payment for home care and out-of-pocket expenditures. Additional information on the characteristics of the population receiving home health care and expenditures for such care is available from the 1977 National Medical Care Expenditure Survey (NMCES).[2]

Need for Home Care in the Elderly Population

While home health care is reimbursed under Medicare for a restricted range of "skilled nursing" and rehabilitation services, survey data show that the greatest need in the elderly population is for personal and supportive care and for assistance with home management activities. The need increases with advancing age and relates to a progressive decrease in functional ability. (For age- and activity-specific estimates of functional disability, see Chapter 4, Tables 4-11 to 4-16).

Functional disability in an elderly person is not necessarily associated with the need for home care. Depending on the level of disability at different ages, some individuals may be able to function adaptively, without assistance, others may require special equipment to overcome the impairment, and others will need assistance from at least one other person to cope with normal daily activities.

Table 7-1 shows estimates, by age, from the 1982 NLTCS, of the type of assistance needed by the functionally disabled elderly to perform specific activities. Loss of independence is highest with regard to bathing (48 percent) and lowest for eating (6 percent). For "getting around inside," "getting in and out of bed," "bathing," and "getting to the bathroom or using the toilet," special equipment provides the assistance needed to perform the activity more frequently than help from another person. For eating and dressing, personal help is the most frequently used type of assistance.

Complete dependency in individual ADL is highest for bathing, at 6 percent of the impaired elderly, followed by dressing and toileting at 2 percent each. Less than 1 percent are totally dependent in other ADL functions.

Home Care Population: Demographic and Social Characteristics

The 1977 NMCES survey showed that for the total population those receiving formal home health care visits were more likely to be women, poor or near poor, and living alone.[2]

Table 7-2 compares estimates from the 1979 NHIS of the population aged 65 and over needing or receiving all forms of home care with the total elderly population for selected demographic and social characteristics. This shows that a lower proportion of whites and a higher proportion of minority races were in the "home care population" than in the general population, and that whereas women comprised 59 percent of the elderly, they accounted for 69 percent of those in need of home care. Sixty-three

Table 7-1. Assistance needed by functionally-disabled elderly, living in the community to perform specified activities of daily living, by age, 1982.

Percentage

Age	Number (thousands)	No assistance	Special equipment only	Personal help only	Special equipment & personal help	Complete dependency	Total
Bathing							
All persons	4962.8	57.9	14.4	13.6	8.4	5.7	100.0
65-69	1083.2	66.2	12.5	10.9	6.4	4.0	100.0
70-74	1087.6	62.4	13.7	11.6	7.9	4.5	100.0
75-79	1046.7	58.5	14.6	12.6	7.9	6.5	100.0
80-84	869.5	52.5	16.8	15.0	9.5	6.2	100.0
85 & over	875.9	46.6	15.0	19.3	11.2	8.0	100.0
Dressing							
All persons	4997.9	80.5	1.3	15.2	1.0	2.1	100.0
65-69	1090.4	80.7	1.4	15.5	1.0	1.5	100.0
70-74	1097.8	82.3	1.2	13.3	1.0	2.3	100.0
75-79	1051.1	80.0	2.0	15.4	0.8	1.8	100.0
80-84	876.2	81.0	1.2	15.2	1.0	1.5	100.0
85 & over	882.5	77.9	0.5	17.1	1.3	3.3	100.0
Getting to bathroom or using toilet							
All persons	5064.3	79.1	10.2	4.1	4.5	2.1	100.0
65-69	1106.1	84.0	6.2	4.2	3.7	1.8	100.0
70-74	1107.4	81.5	9.4	3.9	3.8	1.4	100.0
75-79	1062.8	80.3	9.7	3.2	4.6	2.1	100.0
80-84	884.7	77.3	11.4	4.6	4.7	2.0	100.0
85 & over	903.4	70.2	15.4	4.9	5.7	3.8	100.0

Getting in and out of bed

All persons	5064.0	73.9	13.6	4.6	7.0	0.9	100.0
65-69	1106.8	75.8	11.5	5.2	6.7	0.8	100.0
70-74	1105.6	76.2	13.3	4.1	6.0	0.3	100.0
75-79	1063.6	74.5	12.9	4.4	7.3	0.9	100.0
80-84	884.7	73.4	15.0	3.9	7.1	0.6	100.0
85 & over	904.2	68.4	16.2	5.3	8.3	1.8	100.0

Getting around inside

All persons	5024.6	59.8	28.3	3.0	8.3	0.7	100.0
65-69	1097.5	67.1	22.1	3.2	7.1	0.5	100.0
70-74	1101.5	64.5	25.2	2.5	7.3	0.5	100.0
75-79	1056.8	61.1	27.3	2.9	7.9	0.6	100.0
80-84	880.0	55.8	31.9	2.9	8.4	1.1	100.0
85 & over	888.6	47.5	36.9	3.7	11.1	0.8	100.0

Eating

All persons	5051.1	93.9	0.7	4.6	0.7	0.2	100.0
65-69	1102.6	93.8	1.0	4.4	0.7	0.1	100.0
70-74	1103.5	95.8	0.5	2.9	0.6	0.2	100.0
75-79	1061.6	94.8	0.5	4.3	0.3	0.1	100.0
80-84	881.4	93.9	0.5	4.9	0.6	--	100.0
85 & over	901.9	90.8	0.8	6.7	1.3	0.5	100.0

Note: Sum of percentages may exceed 100.0 because of rounding.

Source: Macken, C. L. 1982 Long-Term Care Survey: National estimates of functional impairments among the elderly living in the community. Office of Research and Demonstrations, Health Care Financing Administration. Working paper, 1984.

145

Table 7-2. Percentage distribution of the total population aged 65 and over, and the home care population aged 65 and over, by selected characteristics, 1979*

| | Percentage with trait | |
Characteristic	Total 65 & over	Home care population aged 65 & over
Race		
White	90.4	86.8
Black	8.8	12.2
Other	0.9	1.1
Sex		
Female	58.8	68.8
Regional location		
Northeast	23.6	25.1
North Central	25.8	22.2
South	33.7	36.2
West	17.0	16.5
Medicaid status		
Program participant	8.4	20.1
Age		
75 & over	36.1	63.0
Living arrangement		
Lives alone	29.3	30.1
Lives with nonrelative	1.4	2.8
Lives with spouse	54.4	37.2
Lives with other relative	14.9	30.0
Number in thousands	(233,359)	(28,176)

* Estimates from the 1979 National Health Interview Survey

Source: Soldo, B.J. A national perspective on the home care population. Presented at the 36th Annual Scientific Meeting of the Gerontological Society of America, San Francisco, November 1983.

percent of the home care population was aged 75 and older compared with 36 percent of the total elderly population, and 20 percent were Medicaid recipients as opposed to 8 percent of all individuals aged 65 and over.

In terms of living arrangements, 29 percent of the elderly were living alone, as were 30 percent of the home care population. Those living with spouses were less likely to be in need of home care (54 percent compared with 37 percent), but whereas 15 percent of the elderly population lived with "other relatives," 30 percent of the home care population had this form of living arrangement.

Table 7-3 illustrates the increasing need for home care with advancing age. While the rate per 1,000 of the home care population in relationship to the total elderly population was 121, it was 70 for those aged 65 to 74 and 211 for those aged 75 and over. In general the proportion of those aged 75 and over needing home care triples compared with those aged 65 to 74. There is a variation from this trend among elderly blacks whose need for home care was twice the rate for whites in the age range 65 to 74 (127 per 1,000 compared with 64 per 1,000). By age 75, the rates had become more comparable at 245 for blacks and 207 for whites.

Women and individuals living in the Northeast and the South reported the need for home care at an earlier age than men and those living in other parts of the country. The elderly rural farm population appeared to have the lowest rates of need for home care compared with the elderly residing in other places. In terms of living arrangements, those living with "nonrelatives" and "other relatives" had a greater need for home care in both the younger and older age groups than individuals living alone or with a spouse.

Finding a relatively low proportion of married persons in the 1979 home care population is consistent with the results of the more recent 1982 NLTCS data. A far higher percentage of men than women are married at advanced ages, and the fact that a spouse is available to assist with ADL and carry out home management activities may result in underreporting of "need for assistance" and functional disability among the elderly male population.

Table 7-4 shows the percentage of the elderly needing personal care assistance and the percentage needing home management assistance by age, sex, and living arrangement. While the percentage increases with age, a relatively low proportion of those living alone at all ages require personal care assistance compared with the percentage needing help with activities related to home management, such as preparing meals and doing laundry. The highest percentage of individuals needing personal care assistance in all age groups was among those living with "other relatives." The low reporting of need for home management assistance by elderly married males is again a reflection of the role played by their spouses.

All available data seem to indicate that the elderly are more likely to lose their ability to live independently when their ADL functioning is impaired and they need assistance with hygiene and other physical care than when IADL functioning is impaired and they need help with home management. The loss of functional ability and need for personal care assistance may increase dependency on a spouse, lead to a change of liv-

Table 7-3. Need for home care for selected population characteristics, by age: prevalence rate per 1,000 persons aged 65 and over, 1979*

Characteristics	Total 65 & over	Age group 65-74	75 & over
Total	121.0	69.9	211.0
Race			
White	116.0	64.0	207.0
Black	168.0	127.0	245.0
Other	148.0	82.0	320.0
Sex			
Male	91.0	55.3	166.6
Female	141.0	81.1	237.2
Region			
Northeast	129.0	78.0	219.0
North Central	104.0	54.0	188.0
South	130.0	80.0	221.0
West	118.0	62.0	216.0
Place of residence			
Central city, SMSA**	123.0	77.0	204.0
SMSA, not central city	113.0	64.0	203.0
Rural, nonfarm	132.0	74.0	230.0
Rural, farm	72.0	25.0	164.0
Living arrangements			
Alone	124.0	77.0	177.0
With non-relative	246.0	132.0	392.0
With spouse	82.0	55.0	163.0
With other relative	243.0	134.0	346.0
Medicaid (last 12 months)			
Yes	292.0	195.0	412.0
No	105.0	60.0	189.0

* Estimates from the 1979 National Health Interview Survey

** Standard Metropolitan Statistical Area

Source: Soldo, B.J. A national perspective on the home care population. Presented at the 36th Annual Scientific Meeting of the Gerontological Society of America, San Francisco, November, 1983.

Table 7-4. Percentage of the elderly needing personal care assistance, and percentage needing home management assistance, by living arrangement, age and sex, 1979 and 1980*

		Living arrangement		
Needing personal care assistance:	Total	Alone	With spouse	With other relatives
Both sexes		Percentage of elderly		
Age:				
65-74	2.2	1.3	2.2	4.3
75-84	5.9	2.6	6.3	11.2
85 & over	17.8	9.6	18.8	25.0
Male				
Age:				
65-74	2.4	1.5	2.5	4.4
75-84	5.5	2.0	6.3	6.1
85 & over	15.2	6.4	18.5	19.8
Female				
Age:				
65-74	2.0	1.3	1.8	4.1
75-84	6.1	2.7	6.3	12.4
85 & over	19.1	10.5	20.2	26.4
Needing home management assistance:				
Both sexes				
Age:				
65-74	4.5	6.8	2.9	8.3
75-84	9.8	11.1	6.5	14.6
85 & over	21.5	24.1	12.7	23.8
Male				
Age:				
65-74	3.0	5.0	2.1	9.6
75-84	6.5	9.2	4.9	12.7
85 & over	15.8	20.0	10.5	23.1
Female				
Age:				
65-74	5.7	7.2	3.8	7.9
75-84	11.9	11.5	9.3	15.1
85 & over	24.7	25.5	21.4	23.8

* Estimates from the 1979 and 1980 National Health Interview Survey.

Source: National Center for Health Statistics: Feller, B.A. Need for care among the noninstitutionalized elderly. Health, United States, 1983 DHHS Pub. No. (PHS)84-1232. Public Health Service, Washington, D.C. U.S. Government Printing Office, December 1984.

Table 7-5. Percentage distribution of sources of home care assistance for elderly persons living in the community, by type of need for those living with a spouse and those living with other relatives, 1979*.

Source of assistance

Type of need:	No Assistance	Informal careproviders only	Formal careproviders only	Formal and informal careproviders	Total
Living with spouse:					
IADL & ADL needs in absence of medical care needs	1.5	80.1	3.3	15.0	100.0
IADL & ADL needs with medical care needs	3.7	41.6	3.8	50.9	100.0
Living with other relative:					
IADL & ADL needs in absence of medical care needs	1.6	89.0	a	8.9	100.0
IADL & ADL needs with medical care needs	a	54.4	a	42.7	100.0

a = Less than 1.5 percent

* Estimates from the 1979 National Health Interview Survey

Source: Soldo, B.J. A national perspective on the home care population. Presented at the 36th Annual Scientific Meeting of the Gerontological Society of America, San Francisco, November, 1983.

150

ing arrangements where other relatives are available for support, or pre-dispose to institutionalization where family, friends, or formal community services are not available.

Informal and Formal Provision of Home Care

All survey data demonstrate that over 70 percent of home care is delivered by family and friends and not by paid providers.[6-9] Detailed analysis of 1979 data show that where an elderly individual was living with a spouse, over 80 percent of care related to ADL and IADL was delivered by informal caregivers and 15 percent by a combination of formal and informal providers. When medical care needs existed in addition to IADL and ADL needs, the proportion of combined formal and informal care rose to over 50 percent. Where an elderly individual was living with relatives other than a spouse, 90 percent of the care related to IADL and ADL needs was delivered informally, and 10 percent by combined formal and informal caregivers. In the presence of medical care needs, the percentage of informal care fell to 54 percent, while 43 percent was delivered by a combination of formal and informal caregivers (see Table 7-5).

Additional data show that the use of formal providers was highest when the elderly person was incontinent: 67 percent of the care was then delivered by formal, or a combination of formal and informal, providers and 33 percent by informal caregivers alone.[7]

Table 7-6 shows 1982 estimates of the distribution of functionally impaired elderly in the community by disability level and the proportion of paid and unpaid help given to individuals at different levels of functioning. Sixty-five percent of the total were only moderately disabled,

Table 7-6. Percentage distribution of functionally-disabled elderly living in the community, by ADL level and by source of assistance, 1982*.

Limitation	Number	All helpers paid	All helpers unpaid	Both paid & unpaid helpers
			Percentage	
Total	4,405,000	5.5	73.9	20.6
IADL only	1,368,000	6.8	81.1	12.1
ADL 1 - 2	1,506,000	6.6	74.9	18.5
ADL 3 - 4	683,000	4.0	68.6	27.4
ADL 5 - 6	849,000	2.5	64.7	32.9

*Data from the 1982 National Long-Term Care Survey

Source: Liu K., Manton K.G., Liu B.M. Home care expenses for the disabled elderly. Health Care Financing Review 7: 2: 51-58, 1985.

their limitations confined to IADL or 1 to 2 ADL activities. At the other extreme, nearly 850,000 individuals, or 19 percent of the disabled elderly, were living in the community with severe limitations of 5 to 6 ADL activities.

Seventy-four percent of all disabled elderly relied entirely on unpaid, informal care, a similar finding to that of the 1979 NHIS. Only 5.5 percent, out of more than 4.4 million persons, relied exclusively on paid care, and this was delivered primarily to those with the lowest disability levels. Those with the most severe limitations had the highest proportion of combined paid and unpaid care.

Both the 1979 and 1982 data indicate that the availability of unpaid, informal care is the key to maintaining the more severely disabled in the community. Table 7-7 gives estimates of the hours per week of informal care provided to disabled elderly persons by sex and marital status and by source of assistance. The highest proportion of care is provided by spouses, 36 percent of the estimated 112 million hours. Thirty-two percent of care is provided by offspring, and a further 22 percent by other relatives. Nearly 80 percent of the 33 million hours of informal care given to disabled married men comes from spouses compared with 67 percent of the 22 million hours of care given to elderly married females. This reflects the high proportion of elderly men who are married, frequently to younger women who are able to assume the caregiving role.

Women without spouses constitute the highest proportion of the elderly population, and they received the largest amount of informal care—over 50 percent was given by offspring and a further 36 percent by other relatives.

Paying for Home Care

An analysis of data from the 1977 NMCES indicated that estimates of sources of payment for home health care were subject to larger measurement error than for other health services and that the results represented the users' perception of who paid for care rather than the true source.[2] The data collected related to "home health" and not to the broader range of home care provision; respondents estimated that 24 percent of home health visits to the elderly involved out-of-pocket expenditures by the individual concerned or by other family members, 22 percent of visits were covered by Medicare, and 13 percent by Medicaid reimbursements.

From the 1982 NLTCS it was estimated that many disabled elderly required in-home care and assistance that was not primarily medical and would not be covered by either public or private third-party insurers. As a result, of approximately 1.2 million disabled elderly persons who indicated that they received formal home care, 41 percent specified themselves as the sole payment source. As with the NMCES, approximately

Table 7-7. Distribution of hours per week of informal care provided to noninstitutionalized, disabled elderly, by source of care, sex and marital status, 1982.

Source of care	Total	Married men	Unmarried men	Married women	Unmarried women
			Number of hours (in millions)		
All helpers	111.9	32.8	10.6	21.8	46.7
Spouse is helper	40.1	25.6	–	14.5	–
Offspring is helper	35.6	4.3	4.0	3.6	23.7
Other relative is helper	25.0	1.4	4.9	2.1	16.6
Nonrelative is helper	11.2	1.5	1.7	1.6	6.4
			Percentage		
All helpers	100.0	100.0	100.0	100.0	100.0
Spouse is helper	35.8	78.0	–	66.5	–
Offspring is helper	31.8	13.1	37.7	16.5	50.7
Other relative is helper	22.3	4.3	46.2	9.6	35.5
Nonrelative is helper	10.0	4.6	16.0	7.3	13.7

*Data from the 1982 National Long-Term Care Survey.

Source: Liu K., Manton K.G., Liu B.M. Home care expenses for noninstitutionalized elderly with ADL and IADL limitations. Working paper, April 1985.

Table 7-8. Sources of payment for home care reported by functionally disabled elderly persons living in the community, receiving paid home care, unadjusted and adjusted for unknown response, 1982.

	All paid helpers		Nursing helpers	
	Percentage			
Payment Source:	Unadjusted	Adjusted	Unadjusted	Adjusted
Sample person only	40.7	55.0	12.8	16.1
Medicare only	8.4	11.4	30.5	38.5
Medicaid only	6.0	8.1	11.7	14.8
Other organization only	4.8	6.5	5.8	7.3
Sample person & Medicare	2.7	3.6	3.1	*3.9
Other private individuals	2.1	2.8	z	z
Medicare & private insurance	2.0	2.7	5.6	7.1
Sample person & other individuals	1.9	2.6	z	z
Sample person & other organization	1.2	1.6	z	z
Medicare & Medicaid	1.0	*1.4	1.8	*2.3
Insurance only	z	z	2.4	*3.0
All other combinations	3.2	4.3	5.4	6.8
Unknown	26.0	0	20.7	0
Number	1,151,762		290,181	

z Less than 1 percent

* Relative standard error greater than 30 percent.

Source: Liu K., Manton K.G., Liu B.M. Home care expenses for the disabled elderly. Health Care Financing Review 7: 2: 51-58, 1985.

26 percent of respondents who stated that paid care was received did not have complete payment source information.[8] Table 7-8 shows the sources of payment for those receiving all forms of paid help and nursing help, both unadjusted and adjusted for the distribution of payment sources in those cases for which complete information was obtained. In 55 percent of cases with complete information, the sample person was the sole payment source for the home care received. In contrast, for care provided by nurses, nurse's aides, and home health aides, 60 percent was reimbursed by third parties. The ratio of nursing helpers to all paid helpers was, however, only 1:4, confirming that a high proportion of the home care required by the disabled elderly is not reimbursed under formal programs. Although Medicare reimbursements accounted for 39 percent of home nursing expenditures in those cases with complete information, the next-highest source of payment was the recipient, at 16 percent, followed by Medicaid at 15 percent of the total.

Table 7-9 shows the characteristics of all disabled elderly, and of those paying privately for home care, in relation to the amount of monthly pay-

Table 7-9. Characteristics of all disabled elderly and of those paying privately for home care, 1982.

Characteristics	All disabled elderly	Private payers				
		Total	Under $15	$15-39	$40-134	$135 & over
Median age	76.0	78.0	77.0	78.0	78.0	81.0
Percent male	34.9	25.1	20.7	28.2	25.4	25.9
Percent married	41.9	31.8	31.0	31.0	36.9	27.5
Median family income	$8,500	8,500	5,500	7,500	9,500	13,000
Percent on Medicaid	14.9	11.5	15.9	*11.5	*10.4	* 8.8
Median ADL score	2.0	2.0	2.0	2.0	2.0	3.0
Percent senile	10.0	9.4	* 3.5	* 3.6	6.7	23.3
Percent incontinent	24.5	27.8	21.1	26.5	29.1	33.4
Percent needing help with meals	6.8	7.6	* 6.6	* 4.9	* 4.7	14.6
Percent needing help with medicine	27.1	27.2	16.3	15.5	21.7	54.7
Percent ever in nursing home	7.6	15.6	13.4	13.2	13.8	21.8
Percent in hospital in past year	37.6	42.5	40.7	38.0	43.2	47.5
Percent use of adult day care	5.2	5.8	*7.3	7.7	*3.9	*4.9
Percent use of outside sources for meals	4.0	7.3	11.8	* 5.6	* 3.9	8.6
Percent with payments for home nursing	6.2	13.9	11.6	8.4	13.3	21.8
Median number of paid helpers per week	0	1.4	1.2	1	1	1
Median number of paid helper days per week	0	2	1	1	2	7
Median number of unpaid helpers per week	1	1	1	1	1	1
Median number of unpaid helper days per week	7	2	2	2	3	2
Number	4,400,000	608,000	136,000	146,000	174,000	153,000

* Relative standard error greater than 30 percent.

Source: Liu K., Manton K.G., Liu B.M. Home care expenses for the disabled elderly. Health Care Financing Review 7: 2: 51-58, 1985.

ment. Private payors were on average older and more likely to be female and unmarried. They also had a lower median number of unpaid helper days per week and higher use of all health care services. A slightly lower proportion of private payors were Medicaid recipients than in the general population of disabled elderly, and they were twice as likely to have made payments for home nursing care.

While the median ADL score for all those paying privately for home care was the same as for all disabled elderly, those paying more than $135 per month had a higher disability score (3 compared with 2) and were twice as likely to be senile and to need help with meals and with taking medicine. The median age was five years higher than for all disabled elderly, 48 percent had had a hospital admission in the past year, and 22 percent had had previous nursing home admissions. They also had three times the rate for all disabled elderly in paying for home nursing. Additional data show that those with high ADL scores (5 to 6) paying over $135 per month accounted for nearly 44 percent of all out-of-pocket payments for home care, even though they comprised only 5.3 percent of the self-paying population. Individuals with IADL disabilities only represented 25 percent of the self-paying population but accounted for just 13 percent of total out-of-pocket expenditures.

Therefore, although higher average monthly payments were associated with higher income, they were also related to the level of assistance needed.

The overall data on payments for home care indicate that for many individuals paid care is substituting for that which is provided to others informally by family and friends. Those with the highest monthly payments for home care had characteristics associated with high rates of nursing home admission, including advanced age, senility, and higher ADL scores. For many of these individuals payments for home care were undoubtedly substituting for institutionalization.

Summary

Home care has assumed increasing importance in the context of the growing number of very elderly persons in the population and the search for lower-cost alternatives to institutional care. Health care and other supportive services in the home may be provided to individuals of all ages in response to illness or disability, with public funding available under a number of programs including Medicare, Medicaid, and Title III of the Older Americans Act. Home health care benefits are also being introduced at an increasing rate by private insurance companies. Nevertheless, studies consistently show that over 70 percent of home care to the sick and functionally disabled is provided by family and friends.

The extent to which care is provided informally to the impaired population in the community depends on the level of functional disability, the presence or absence of medical care needs, and the availability of a spouse or other family member willing to provide such care.

Although a high proportion of functionally disabled elderly persons in the community are only moderately impaired, nearly 20 percent are being maintained at home with severe limitations. The ratio of formal to informal care increases in the presence of medical care needs and is highest when the individual is incontinent. Elderly women receive a higher proportion of home care than men but, where most home care for elderly men is provided by a spouse, children or other relatives provide most of the informal home care for elderly women.

Although data on private payments for home care are subject to greater measurement error than those for other health expenditures, many impaired individuals in all income groups pay privately to supplement or to substitute for the care that might be provided by informal caregivers or under formal programs. The recent national study of functionally disabled elderly persons in the community showed that where complete information was available, in over 50 percent of cases the individual concerned was the only payment source for the home care received. Although the majority of private payors suffered minor impairments and paid relatively modest amounts for assistance with home management activities, a high proportion of total private expenditures was accounted for by the most severely impaired. In addition to high levels of functional disability, those with the highest private payments showed other characteristics of individuals who are at high risk of institutionalization: advanced age, severe cognitive impairment, and previous nursing home admissions.

Since a high proportion of severely disabled persons are being maintained in the community on a long-term basis, it must be concluded that home care is instrumental in reducing the overall rate of institutionalization. The informal care provided by family and friends is supplemented by formal programs for eligible individuals, but a high proportion of the home care received is paid for privately by the recipients. In the case of the most disabled, home care may be deferring the time for admission to a nursing home, and for those lacking family and other voluntary support the cost may be equal to or higher than institutional care.

For further details and discussions of publicly funded home and community based programs, see Chapters 8 to 11.

REFERENCES

1. Palmer H. C. Home care. In Vogel R. J. and Palmer H. C. (eds), Long-Term Care: Perspectives from Research and Demonstrations. Health Care Financing Administration. U.S. Government Printing Office: 1983.
2. Berk M. L., Bernstein A. Use of home health services: some findings from the

National Medical Care Expenditure Survey. Home Health Care Services Quarterly 6: 1: 13–23, 1985.

3. Mundinger M. O'N. Home Care Controversy: too little, too late, too costly. Aspen Books, Rockville, Md. and London, 1983.

4. Cohen, J. Public programs financing long-term care. In Vol. IV, Project to Analyze Existing Long-Term Care Data, The Urban Institute, Washington, D.C. 1983.

5. Lenz E. A. Financing of home health services. Presented at the Complex Cube of Long-Term Care, National Working Conference, Sponsored by the American Health Planning Association and the Veterans Administration, September 23–26, 1984.

6. Doty P. Family care of the elderly: is it declining? Can public policy promote it? Office of Legislation and Policy, Health Care Financing Administration, (working paper) 1984.

7. Soldo B. J. A national perspective on the home care population. Paper presented at the 36th Annual Scientific Meeting of the Gerontological Society of America, San Francisco, November 1983.

8. Liu K, Manton, K. G., Liu B. M. Home care expenses for the disabled elderly. Health Care Financing Review 7: 2: 51–58, 1985.

9. Manton K. G. and Liu K. The future growth of the long-term care population: projections based on the 1977 National Nursing Home Survey and the 1982 Long-Term Care Survey. Presented at the Third National Leadership Conference on Long-Term Care Issues, Washington, D.C., March 7–9, 1984.

10. Williams J., Gaumer G., Cella M. Home health services: an industry in transition. ABT Associates Inc., Washington, D.C. Prospective Payment Demonstration Contract No. 500-84-0021 HCFA. Prepared for the Health Care Financing Administration, May 3, 1984.

11. National Center for Health Statistics. Feller B.A. Need for care among the noninstitutionalized elderly. Health, United States, 1983. DHHS Pub. No. (PHS)84-1232. Public Health Service, Washington, D.C. U.S. Government Printing Office, December 1983.

12. Macken C. L. 1982 Long-Term Care Survey: National estimates of functional impairments among the elderly living in the community. Office of Research and Demonstrations, Health Care Financing Administration, (working paper), 1984.

13. Macken C. L. Descriptive profile of the functionally impaired aged living in the community: findings from the 1982 Long-Term Care Survey. Office of Research and Demonstrations, Health Care Financing Administration, draft report, 1985.

8

Home Health Care:
The Reimbursement System

Visiting nurse associations (VNA's) and public health nursing developed in New England, New York, and other major cities at the end of the 19th century. They provided services primarily for the sick poor; VNA's had adult care as a focus, and public health nursing emphasized maternal and child care. The Metropolitan Life Insurance Company started a major home health care program in 1909 for its policyholders in New York City; the objective was to restrict the number of claims by reducing mortality and promoting health. This program expanded to cover many towns in the United States and Canada, affiliating with 850 VNA's and directly employing over 700 nurses. Peak utilization was in 1931 but, subsequently, the program declined and was discontinued in 1952. Hospital-based home care for the local community was developed by hospitals such as Montefiore in New York, which initiated a program in 1946 to provide posthospital care in the home.[2]

Before Medicare, most home care was delivered by VNA's to the chronically ill who needed subacute nursing care, with payment made privately on a sliding scale. Nursing was the primary and often the only service offered.[2]

The first federal funding for home care came with Medical Assistance for the Aged, the Kerr-Mills legislation of 1960. In addition to nursing coverage it allowed medical vendor payments for "home health aides," similar in function to hospital aides, who were permitted to provide light housekeeping in the patient's room as well as personal care. This created a new category of home care personnel, which later came to be included under health insurance benefits.[2]

The introduction of Medicare and Medicaid in 1966 brought changes in the financing of health care and had the potential for introducing a range of alternatives in health care provision, particularly in the field of home care. In the event a strictly "medical model" was adopted under Medicare, with reimbursement limited to skilled nursing, medical, and rehabilitation services delivered to the homebound under a physician-prescribed plan of care. An early Medicare bill provided coverage for homemakers in the home care benefits, but these were replaced by home health aide services, thereby emphasizing that Medicare is a medical benefit for the sick and not a maintenance program for the disabled elderly.[2]

By contrast, Medicaid has the potential for providing a wider range of personal and supportive home care services; however, coverage and eligibility are determined by the individual states, and there is substantial variation in service provision.

Medicare

Home health services under Medicare are defined as those provided or arranged for by a home health agency, under the supervision of a physician, and delivered in an individual's home.

Medicare-covered home health services consist of: part-time or intermittent nursing care provided by, or under the supervision of, a registered nurse; physical, occupational, and speech therapy; medical social services under the direction of a physician; part-time or intermittent services of a home health aide who has completed approved training; medical supplies and the use of medical appliances; and in the case of hospital-based agencies, medical services provided by interns and residents in approved teaching programs.[3]

Medicare home health services may be provided only to homebound beneficiaries who are under the care of a physician and in need of either skilled nursing services on an intermittent basis or of physical, occupational, or speech therapy.

Home health agencies, like skilled nursing facilities, are paid under Medicare on the basis of retrospectively determined reasonable costs. In 1969 reimbursement criteria issued to fiscal intermediaries led to more restricted coverage than when Medicare was first introduced, and in 1973 a ceiling on reimbursements was set at the 80th percentile of reasonable costs.[4] In 1973, however, coverage for home health services under Medicare was extended to disabled persons and those with end-stage renal disease; since that time, there has been a steady growth in Medicare reimbursements, followed by an increase in the number of participating agencies.

The major impetus to growth and change in recent years has come from the Omnibus Reconciliation Act of 1980. Its implementation in 1981 liberalized the Medicare home health care benefit and made provisions for greater participation by proprietary home health agencies.

In order to participate in the Medicare program, it is required that agencies be primarily engaged in the provision of skilled nursing and other therapeutic services; that policies be established by a professional group associated with the agency to govern the provision of services; that policies provide for the supervision of services by a physician or registered nurse; and that the agency be licensed in accordance with state and local laws where home health care licensing laws exist. Before July 1981,

only nonprofit organizations or those licensed by state law could participate in the program. Consequently, proprietary agencies in states without
licensing laws were excluded from Medicare certification. Under current
law, proprietary agencies in such states may participate if they meet the
rest of the participation requirements.[3] An additional change, implemented in 1981, is that proprietary agencies are now allowed to contract
with other agencies for the provision of services.

Home health care services are reimburseable under both Part A, the
hospital insurance program, and Part B, the supplementary medical
insurance program. When the home health benefit was first introduced
into the Medicare program, there was a limit of 100 visits per benefit
period under Part A and 100 visits per calendar year under part B. Prior
hospitalization or skilled nursing facility stay was also required. Part B
had no prior hospitalization requirement and could be used when coverage was exhausted under Part A.

Under the Omnibus Reconciliation Act, all limits on the number of
visits, the need for prior hospitalization, and the Part B deductible were
eliminated. Services are now paid for under Part A unless the beneficiary
is not enrolled under the Part A program.

The 1980 amendments were intended to increase utilization of the
Medicare home health benefit, and the predicted growth has now been
further stimulated by the introduction of prospective payment for hospital care, with the incentive for earlier discharge of Medicare patients
following an episode of acute illness.

There presently are no deductible or coinsurance charges for home
health visits, but the recent overall increase in Medicare expenditures at
a time of severe constraints on public expenditures has led to scrutiny of
the home health reimbursement system and proposals for changes to control costs.

Prior to July 1983, medical supplies and equipment, classified as durable medical equipment (DME), were available under both Parts A and
B of Medicare, without copayments or deductibles to home health beneficiaries, when the equipment was supplied directly or by arrangement
with a participating home health agency. Since July 1984, home health
agencies have been reimbursed at 80 percent of "reasonable costs," with
20 percent copayment by the patient.

Proposals have now been put forward for copayments for home health
visits,[5] while in the longer term a study is underway to test the feasibility
of introducing prospective payment for home health care to provide
incentives for "efficiency and cost control."[4]

Medicaid

Medicaid home health services must be made available to all Medicaid
recipients eligible for skilled nursing facility care but, since 1976, federal
guidelines have stipulated that home health benefits should not be lim-

ited through use of a "skilled care" requirement. Eligibility has never depended on prior hospitalization, and the number of visits is not limited.

Medicaid regulations specify only that home health services must be provided in the patient's home, on the orders of a physician, with a plan of care written by the physician and reviewed every 60 days. Services covered are nursing (not necessarily "skilled") provided on a part-time or intermittent basis by a home health agency or a registered nurse, oriented to acceptable clinical and administrative record-keeping by a health department nurse; home health aide services provided by a home health agency; and medical supplies, equipment, and appliances suitable for home use. These are the only home health services that must be offered under Medicaid, but states may expand the range of services to include physical, occupational, and speech therapy and audiology services if they wish.[3]

While the potential for home health provision appears to be greater under Medicaid than Medicare, each state determines the scope and range of services to be made available once federal minimum criteria have been met. States may restrict coverage for those who are eligible for Medicaid home health services in a number of ways. Nearly three quarters of states restrict nursing care by requiring prior authorization, physician oversight, or by imposing limits on the number of visits. Some states impose severe limitations on home health aide service, while physical, occupational, and speech therapy are limited or not covered in the majority of states.[4]

All home health agencies certified by Medicare are automatically eligible for Medicaid certification, but many agencies do not choose to treat Medicaid clients. By 1984, eighteen states had instituted some form of prospective payment system for home health services, and this and other reimbursement structures under Medicaid are frequently unattractive to home health agencies.[4]

Medicaid is the payor of last resort for those not eligible for Medicare or other insurance benefits, and this fact contributes in part to a lower proportion of total Medicaid program expenditures being made for home health care compared with the Medicare program.

Services provided under the Medicaid "personal care option" are not reported under payments for "home health," nor are other home and community support programs being developed under Section 2176 of the 1981 Omnibus Budget Reconciliation Act or other Medicaid provisions (see Chapters 9 and 11).

DATA SOURCES

Sources of information for the tables presented in this chapter are as follows:

The Health Care Financing Administration, Office of Statistics and Data Management, provides reimbursement and utilization information for Medicare, with limited data relating to beneficiary characteristics such as age. The Office of Financial and Actuarial analysis provides Medicaid data on total payments by service and by recipient category.

Data on the characteristics of home health agencies are available from the Medicare and Medicaid Automated Certification System.

A recent survey conducted for the Select Committee on Aging of the House of Representatives had a low response rate, but it provides additional information on the characteristics of Medicare-certified home health agencies and the clients they serve.[6]

Medicare: Reimbursements and Utilization

The restrictive reimbursement criteria issued to fiscal intermediaries in 1969 led to a fall in total Medicare reimbursements for home health services and a substantial decline in the number of home health visits between 1969 and 1972 (see Table 8-1). In addition, the proportion of total Medicare reimbursements going for home care fell to less than 1 percent during this period. Since the extension of Medicare benefits to the disabled and those with end-stage renal disease in 1973, there has been a substantial increase in reimbursements and visits every year. The rate of increase declined between 1977 and 1980 but has accelerated to nearly 20 percent a year since 1981. In 1983 reimbursements for home health services represented nearly 3 percent of the Medicare total compared with 2 percent in 1980.

The utilization of Medicare home health services increased in terms of the number of persons served, number of visits, and visits per enrollee every year between 1975 and 1983 (see Table 8-2). There has been a recent major increase in the number of visits per person served; the average for 1983 was 21 percent higher than in 1980, while the average cost per visit rose 30 percent during the same period. Table 8-3 shows that there was a progressive increase in the mean and median number of home health visits between 1975 and 1982, as the proportion of beneficiaries receiving between 1 and 10 visits declined and the proportion receiving more than 50 visits increased progressively. These data indicate that an increasing proportion of individuals are receiving Medicare-reimbursed home health care services, some on a longer-term basis than previously.

Total Medicare home health charges increased 68 percent for the United States as a whole between 1981 and 1983, with the highest rate of increase being in the South and the West (see Table 8-4). By contrast, the average charge per visit increased by only 20 percent, ranging from 16 percent in the South to 21 percent in all other regions. The variation by state is shown in Table 8-5: total charges increased by over 150 percent

Table 8-1. Total Medicare reimbursements, reimbursements for home health services, number of home health visits and percentage change, 1969-1983.

Year	Total Medicare reimbursements (In millions)	Home health reimbursements (In millions)	Percentage of reimbursements	Visits (In thousands)	Percentage change
1969	6,284	78	1.3	8,500	-
1970	6,772	62	0.9	6,000	-29.9
1971	7,487	57	0.8	4,800	-20.5
1972	8,217	66	0.8	5,200	9.2
1973	9,638	93	1.0	6,400	22.4
1974	11,920	144	1.2	8,200	23.4
1975	14,749	217	1.5	10,900	37.0
1976	17,940	295	1.7	13,500	26.4
1977	21,109	367	1.8	15,600	16.2
1978	24,424	427	1.8	17,100	11.4
1979	28,340	518	1.9	19,200	13.3
1980	33,905	662	2.0	22,400	12.4
1981	44,754	1,008	2.3	26,200	15.9
1982	52,371	1,249	2.4	31,300	19.5
1983	59,861	1,669	2.8	37,300	19.2

Comparative data for years prior to 1969 are not available.

Source: Health Care Financing Administration, Bureau of Data Management and Strategy, unpublished data 1983.

Table 8-2. Medicare utilization of home health services, selected calendar years, 1975-1983.

Calendar year	Persons served (In thousands)	Home health visits (In millions)	Visits per 1,000 enrollees	Visits per person served	Average charge per visit
1975	500	10.8	431	21.6	$20
1977	700	15.8	597	22.5	25
1979	870	20.0	717	22.9	30
1980	960	22.6	792	23.4	33
1981	1,080	26.2	902	24.3	36
1982	1,190	31.3	1,060	26.3	40
1983*	1,320	37.3	1,242	28.3	43
Annual percentage increase 1975-1983	12.9	16.8	14.1	2.9	10.0

* Estimate

Source: Health Care Financing Administration, Bureau of Data Management and Strategy: Health Care Spending Bulletin, No. 85-01, February 1985.

Table 8-3. Medicare: percentage distribution of persons served, by number of home health visits, selected calendar years, 1975, 1980, 1982.

| | | Year | |
Number of visits	1975	1980	1982
Total	100.0	100.0	100.0
1-4	24.1	21.2	20.0
5-9	20.2	20.2	19.2
10-19	22.1	22.6	22.3
20-29	11.3	11.7	12.0
30-39	6.5	6.9	7.2
40-49	4.3	4.5	4.8
50-99	8.6	9.3	9.8
100 and over	2.9	3.6	4.8
Mean	21.6	23.4	26.3
Median	12.5	13.8	14.9

Source: Health Care Financing Administration, Bureau of Data Management and Strategy: Health Care Spending Bulletin, No. 85-01, February 1985.

in Arizona, Nevada, and Tennessee but by less than 18 percent in North Dakota and South Dakota. The high rate of increase in states such as Arizona and Tennessee is associated with the recent major growth in the number of home health agencies, most of which are proprietary. The increase in total charges was not necessarily associated with substantially higher costs per visit. Arizona, for instance, had only an 11-percent increase in average visit charge, demonstrating that the increase in total charges was a reflection of a major increase in home health visits.

There was an overall 40-percent increase in the number of home health visits between 1981 and 1983; the South and West had the highest rate of increase and the Northeast the lowest (see Table 8-6). The number of nursing visits increased by 33 percent, the lowest increase being in the North Central region and the highest in the South. As shown in Table 8-7, the highest increase in total visits and nursing visits—over 100 percent—occurred in Arizona, Nevada, Oklahoma, and Tennessee. By contrast, there was a net decline in the total number of visits in North Dakota and South Dakota and of nursing visits in New Hampshire and Vermont.

Medicare-Certified Home Health Agencies

At the beginning of the Medicare program, there were 1,850 home health agencies, most of which were VNA's and local public health departments. There was a 21-percent increase in the number of home health agencies

Table 8-4. Medicare: home health agency charges, average charge per visit and percentage change, by census region and division, 1981 and 1983.

	Total charges (In thousands)		Percentage change 1981-1983	Average charge		Percentage change 1981-1983
	1981	1983		1981	1983	
United States	988,682	1,623,563	68	35.90	43.10	20
Census region & divisions:						
Northeast	291,322	443,758	52	31.72	38.44	21
New England	72,517	117,478	62	25.36	31.24	19
Middle Atlantic	218,804	326,280	49	34.07	41.92	23
North central	194,083	302,451	56	34.93	42.37	21
East North Central	131,562	200,655	53	38.22	45.65	19
West North Central	62,521	101,795	63	29.36	36.94	26
South	333,173	615,430	85	37.73	43.85	16
South Atlantic	169,994	288,093	69	37.65	41.82	11
East South Central	79,956	160,162	100	36.69	43.21	18
West South Central	83,223	167,175	100	38.44	48.66	27
West	149,955	261,897	75	44.32	53.52	21
Mountain	26,519	48,209	82	35.86	44.89	25
Pacific	123,435	213,688	73	46.70	56.02	20

Source: Health Care Financing Administration, Bureau of Data Management and Strategy, unpublished data, June 1984.

Table 8-5. Medicare: home health agency charges, average charge per visit and percentage change, by state, 1981 and 1983.

State	Total charges		Percentage change 1981-1983	Average charge per visit		Percentage change 1981-1983
	1981	1983		1981	1983	
	(In thousands)					
United States	968,682	1,623,563	67.6	35.9	43.1	20.1
Alabama	21,344	31,847	49.2	35.7	42.2	18.2
Alaska	143	285	99.3	42.3	65.6	55.0
Arizona	2,797	8,407	200.6	44.0	48.9	11.1
Arkansas	10,690	15,783	47.6	39.9	47.7	19.5
California	94,922	169,956	79.0	48.3	57.5	19.1
Colorado	11,180	17,661	58.0	37.6	50.0	33.1
Connecticut	19,754	30,281	53.3	27.6	33.0	19.7
Delaware	2,082	4,579	119.9	24.1	29.6	23.0
District of Columbia	2,342	4,133	76.5	35.4	42.9	21.4
Florida	91,637	155,620	69.8	39.0	43.4	11.3
Georgia	21,985	34,758	58.1	45.1	50.2	11.2
Hawaii	1,975	3,176	60.8	43.7	58.1	33.1
Idaho	3,186	4,479	40.6	36.0	39.3	9.2
Illinois	50,768	74,685	47.1	43.1	50.8	18.0
Indiana	8,482	14,636	72.6	28.5	35.8	25.4
Iowa	5,540	7,663	38.3	20.2	25.1	24.5
Kansas	6,731	12,966	92.6	27.5	34.1	24.3
Kentucky	8,632	13,312	54.2	34.8	39.9	14.5
Louisiana	18,486	33,753	82.6	35.0	45.8	30.9
Maine	4,515	5,791	28.3	29.1	32.6	12.1
Maryland	15,773	24,696	56.6	39.7	46.3	16.6
Massachusetts	36,144	63,393	75.4	25.4	30.1	18.4
Michigan	29,259	52,522	79.5	44.5	50.5	13.5
Minnesota	8,020	9,804	22.2	33.4	42.3	26.8
Mississippi	26,817	49,921	86.2	37.7	42.4	12.5
Missouri	35,940	62,106	72.8	31.4	39.0	24.3
Montana	1,242	2,201	77.2	29.3	34.9	19.2
Nebraska	3,848	6,430	67.1	33.2	40.4	21.7
Nevada	1,269	3,312	161.0	39.7	49.0	23.5
New Hampshire	3,181	4,070	27.9	24.7	31.5	27.8
New Jersey	45,021	59,974	33.2	31.0	36.2	16.7
New Mexico	3,529	6,511	84.5	37.6	45.9	21.9
New York	90,441	131,685	45.6	38.3	48.2	25.8
North Carolina	11,493	23,558	105.0	30.3	35.1	16.1
North Dakota	1,356	1,593	17.5	24.9	33.9	36.2
Ohio	30,061	39,793	32.4	33.7	41.7	23.7
Oklahoma	5,951	14,027	135.7	42.2	49.7	17.8
Oregon	10,127	15,389	52.0	42.7	53.4	25.1
Pennsylvania	83,342	134,622	61.5	32.0	39.7	24.2
Rhode Island	6,402	10,940	70.9	29.0	33.8	16.4
South Carolina	9,736	16,164	66.0	34.4	35.2	2.5
South Dakota	1,087	1,234	13.5	23.8	34.7	46.1
Tennessee	23,164	65,082	181.0	37.2	45.1	21.2
Texas	47,364	103,291	118.1	39.9	49.6	24.3
Utah	1,636	3,489	113.3	24.2	31.9	31.6
Vermont	2,522	3,002	19.0	23.9	27.8	16.3
Virginia	8,224	14,524	76.6	33.6	34.3	2.3
Washington	16,268	24,382	49.9	41.5	48.6	17.2
West Virginia	6,723	10,061	49.7	30.8	35.9	16.4
Wisconsin	12,992	19,019	46.4	31.1	36.6	17.8
Wyoming	1,059	1,982	87.2	28.1	34.0	21.1

Source: Health Care Financing Administration, Bureau of Data Management and Strategy, unpublished data, June 1984.

Table 8-6. Medicare: all home health visits, nursing visits and percentage change, by census region and division, 1981 and 1983.

	All visits 1981 1983 (In thousands)		Percentage change 1981-1983	Nursing visits 1981 1983 (In thousands)		Percentage change 1981-83
United States	25,773	36,284	40.1	13,162	17,511	33
Census Region & Divisions:						
Northeast	8,853	11,325	28	4,384	5,348	31
New England	2,700	3,232	20	1,312	1,474	12
Middle Atlantic	6,153	7,631	24	3,072	3,724	22
North Central	5,280	7,004	33	3,047	3,698	21
East North Central	3,382	4,367	29	2,015	2,395	19
West North Central	1,998	2,637	32	1,003	1,303	26
South	8,328	13,362	60	4,139	6,325	53
South Atlantic	4,333	6,628	53	2,044	2,966	45
East South Central	2,005	3,457	72	987	1,594	61
West South Central	1,991	3,276	65	1,109	1,764	59
West	3,207	4,593	43	1,589	2,140	35
Mountain	702	1,031	47	388	538	39
Pacific	2,506	3,562	42	1,201	1,602	33

Source: Health Care Financing Administration, Bureau of Data Management and Strategy, unpublished data, June 1984.

between 1966 and 1970, but the changes in administrative interpretation of the Medicare benefit after 1969 that led to a decline in total reimbursements (see above) also led to a net fall of 2 percent in the number of participating home health agencies between 1970 and 1975. Since then, the number of participating agencies has shown continuous growth.

The extent to which Medicare-certified home health agencies depend on Medicare funding is shown in Table 8-8. This indicates that 80 percent of revenues are from funds provided under federal programs, 67 percent of which come from Medicare.[6] These figures represent the findings from a national survey of home health agencies that had only an 18-percent response rate and may be biased by a disproportionately low response rate from proprietary agencies, which have been assuming an increasing proportion of the home health care market.

The composition of the home health industry has been changing since the implementation of Medicare, but the change has accelerated since 1981. The actual number of voluntary and public sector home health

Table 8-7. Medicare: all home health visits, nursing visits and percentage change, by state, 1981 and 1983.

	All visits 1981 1983 (In thousands)		Percentage change 1981-1983	Nursing visits 1981 1983 (In thousands)		Percentage change 1981-1983
United States	25,773	36,284	40.1	13,162	17,511	33.0
Alabama	569	737	29.5	270	327	21.1
Alaska	3	4	33.3	2	2	0.0
Arizona	59	156	164.4	35	80	128.6
Arkansas	260	323	24.2	139	148	6.5
California	1,869	2,757	47.5	863	1,200	39.0
Colorado	295	354	20.0	156	182	16.7
Connecticut	711	923	29.8	294	353	20.1
Delaware	82	148	80.5	35	63	80.0
District of Columbia	66	101	53.0	34	47	38.2
Florida	2,274	3,511	54.4	979	1,475	50.7
Georgia	455	648	42.4	197	270	37.1
Hawaii	41	49	19.5	24	27	12.5
Idaho	75	99	32.0	43	50	16.3
Illinois	1,160	1,447	24.7	628	771	22.8
Indiana	285	399	40.0	173	221	27.7
Iowa	271	306	12.9	146	157	7.5
Kansas	242	382	57.9	117	162	38.5
Kentucky	222	305	37.4	122	140	14.8
Louisiana	458	654	42.8	176	250	42.0
Maine	150	172	14.7	89	91	2.2
Maryland	385	523	35.8	195	259	32.8
Massachusetts	1,394	2,053	47.3	678	875	29.1
Michigan	649	1,035	59.5	388	552	42.3
Minnesota	233	234	0.4	114	122	7.0
Mississippi	637	1,049	64.7	317	502	58.4
Missouri	1,050	1,488	41.7	522	705	35.1
Montana	40	63	57.5	25	40	60.0
Nebraska	103	146	41.7	74	105	41.9
Nevada	31	64	106.5	14	29	107.1
New Hampshire	128	131	2.3	76	75	-1.3
New Jersey	1,401	1,633	16.6	468	572	22.2
New Mexico	89	138	55.1	46	71	54.3
New York	2,253	2,664	18.2	1,032	1,194	15.7
North Carolina	355	589	65.9	187	269	43.9
North Dakota	54	46	-14.8	30	28	-6.7
Ohio	880	947	7.6	558	535	-4.1
Oklahoma	137	284	107.3	88	181	105.7
Oregon	219	275	25.6	130	154	18.5
Pennsylvania	2,499	3,334	33.4	1,572	1,968	25.2
Rhode Island	212	307	44.8	118	163	38.1
South Carolina	270	435	61.1	169	254	50.3
South Dakota	45	36	-20.0	30	23	23.3
Tennessee	577	1,366	136.7	278	625	124.8
Texas	1,120	2,010	79.5	694	1,181	70.2
Utah	62	101	62.9	42	59	40.5
Vermont	104	107	2.9	57	56	-1.8
Virginia	241	413	71.4	128	192	50.0
Washington	374	477	27.5	182	219	20.3
West Virginia	205	260	26.8	120	138	15.0
Wisconsin	408	538	31.9	268	316	17.9
Wyoming	35	53	51.4	19	26	36.8

Source: Health Care Financing Administration, Bureau of Data Management and and Strategy, unpublished data, June 1984.

Table 8-8. Revenue sources of Medicare-certified home health agencies, 1982.*

Revenue source	Average revenues in 1982	Percentage of total revenues
Total	$740,931	100.0
Medicare	494,196	67.0
Medicaid	70,045	9.0
Private health insurance (including Blue Cross)	49,783	6.5
Title XX	13,174	2.0
Title III OAA	6,646	1.0
Veterans' Administration	3,534	0.5
United Way	20,590	3.0
Private gifts/Contributions	7,352	1.0
Private pay	42,619	5.5
Grants	32,992	4.5

* As represented by a response rate of 18 percent to a survey of Medicare-certified home health agencies.

Source: Building a long-term care policy: home care data and implications. Report of the Subcommittee on Long-Term Care of the Select Committee on Aging, House of Representatives. Comm. Pub. No. 98-484, December 1984.

agencies showed only a slight decline between 1967 and 1983, but their share of the Medicare home health market dropped from 83 percent in 1972 to 42 percent in 1983 as the number of proprietary agencies and their market share increased.[4]

Table 8-9 shows the increase in the number of home health agencies, by auspices, between 1972 and 1982 and between 1982 and 1985. From 1982 to March 1, 1985, there was a 170-percent increase in the number of proprietary agencies (from 628 to 1,695).

With the financial incentive for earlier discharge of Medicare patients under prospective reimbursement for hospital care, an increase in hospital-based agencies might be predicted. In fact, between 1982 and 1985 there was a 92-percent increase in the number of such agencies (from 507 to 972). The number of nursing home, skilled nursing facility-based agencies also increased during the same period, from 32 to 168. This increase in the number of institutional-based agencies is likely to continue.

The change in the distribution of persons receiving home health services, by type of agency, between 1975 and 1982 is shown in Table 8-10. There was a progressive decline in the proportion served by VNA's and other voluntary and government agencies and an increase in the proportion served by proprietary and private nonprofit agencies. In addition, the average number of visits per person served and average charge per

Table 8-9. Distribution of Medicare-certified home health agencies by auspices, and percentage change over time, 1972, 1982 and 1985.

Type of ownership	1972		1982		March 1, 1985		Percentage change	
	Number	Percent	Number	Percent	Number	Percent	1972-82	1982-85
VNA	531	24.0	517	14.2	527	9.7	-2.6	19.0
Combination	55	2.5	59	1.6	60	1.1	7.3	1.7
Official health agency	1,255	56.7	1,211	33.3	1,225	22.5	-3.5	1.2
Rehabilitation facility-based	11	0.5	16	0.4	21	0.4	45.5	31.3
Hospital-based	231	10.4	507	13.9	972	17.8	119.5	91.7
SNF-based	7	0.3	32	0.9	168	3.1	357.1	425.0
Proprietary	43	1.9	628	17.3	1,695	31.1	1360.5	170.0
Private non-profit	*	*	632	17.4	761	14.0	--	20.4
Other and unclassified	79	3.6	37	1.0				
Totals	2,212	100.0	3,639	100.0	5,447	100.0	64.5	50.0

* No listing

Source: Williams J., Gaumer G. and Cella M. Home health services: an industry in transition, ABT Associates Inc., Washington, D.C. Prospective Payment Demonstration Contract No. 500-84-0021 HCFA. Prepared for the Health Care Financing Administration, May 3, 1984, and Health Care Financing Administration, Division of Data and Program Analysis, April 1985.

visit and per person served was also higher for proprietary and private nonprofit agencies than for VNA or other voluntary or government agencies.

Home Health Agencies: Services Provided

Table 8-11 shows the distribution of Medicare-certified home health agencies providing different types of services in 1984. All agencies offered skilled nursing (a requirement for Medicare certification), 94 percent offered home health aide, and 83 percent offered physical therapy. These were also the services most likely to be provided by agency staff, with 99 percent employing nurses, 84 percent home health aides, and 52 percent physical therapists. Pharmaceutical services were offered by only 6 percent of agencies.

The distribution of persons served by type of home health service, from 1974 to 1980, is shown in Table 8-12. While the percentage receiving nursing care has remained constant during this period, the percentage receiving home health aide services increased from 24 percent in 1974 to 36 percent in 1980, at an annual compound rate of growth of 24 percent. There was also an annual 22-percent increase in the proportion receiving physical therapy and a 32-percent increase in the growth of other services, including speech and occupational therapy and medical social services.

In terms of home health agency staffing, as shown in Table 8-13, the average number of full-time equivalent registered nurses employed by home health agencies was higher in voluntary, government, and other nonprofit agencies than in proprietary and private nonprofit agencies, while the average number of licensed practical nurses was highest in proprietary agencies. The average number of all full-time equivalent staff was lowest for government agencies, followed by private nonprofit and proprietary agencies.

A recent survey of Medicare-certified home health agencies indicates that approximately 30 percent of all home health agency staff are contracted and not directly employed.[6]

Medicare Home Health Service Recipients

The home health agency survey cited above indicated a decline in the proportion of Medicare home health beneficiaries aged 65 and over, from 93 percent of all home health beneficiaries in 1978 to 75 percent in 1982. It also indicated that a disproportionate number of the average agency's clients were female (64 percent) and black (14 percent).[6]

Table 8-14 shows comparable data for 1977 and 1980 on Medicare home health recipients aged 65 and over. There were increases for all age groups in terms of the total number of users, the number of users per 1,000 enrollees, visits, and visits per 1,000 enrollees.

Table 8-10. Medicare: percentage distribution of persons receiving home health visits and charges, by type of agency, 1975, 1980 and 1982.

	All agencies	Visiting Nurse Association	Combination government and voluntary	Government	Hospital based	Proprietary	Private non-profit	Other
Persons served								
1975	100.0	46.4	4.2	22.5	11.5	3.8	10.1	1.5
1980	100.0	39.4	1.7	18.1	11.9	6.4	21.1	1.4
1982	100.0	36.8	1.5	16.9	13.2	10.6	19.5	1.4
Visits								
1975	100.0	42.2	3.0	21.6	10.7	5.6	15.3	1.6
1980	100.0	37.6	1.4	15.9	10.8	7.1	25.8	1.4
1982	100.0	35.8	1.2	14.3	11.4	12.3	23.7	1.4
Visit charges								
1975	100.0	38.0	3.1	18.6	13.5	6.5	18.7	1.6
1980	100.0	33.2	1.3	12.8	12.5	8.2	30.4	1.4
1982	100.0	32.0	1.2	11.4	14.3	14.1	25.7	1.4

Average number of visits per persons served								
1975	21.6	19.7	15.5	20.7	20.1	32.0	32.8	23.8
1980	23.4	22.4	18.7	20.6	21.2	25.7	28.8	23.6
1982	26.3	25.5	20.6	22.3	22.6	30.5	31.8	26.0
Average visit charges per person served								
1975	$424	$348	$311	$351	$497	$731	$786	$445
1980	767	647	605	543	809	981	1,109	755
1982	1,052	913	818	713	1,136	1,393	1,384	1,042
Average charge per visit								
1975	$20	$18	$20	$17	$25	$23	$24	$19
1980	33	29	32	26	38	38	39	32
1982	40	36	40	32	50	46	43	40

Source: Health Care Financing Administration, Bureau of Data Management and Strategy: Health Care Spending Bulletin, No. 85-01. February, 1985.

Table 8-11. Number of home health agencies providing in-home services, by type of service, and by staff or other arrangements, January 1984.

Type of service offered**	Number	Percentage		
		Total	By staff	By arrangement
All home health agencies*	4,284			
Skilled nursing	4,270	100.0	98.6	1.4
Physical therapy	3,546	83.0	52.0	31.0
Occupational therapy	2,104	49.3	28.9	20.4
Speech therapy	2,793	65.4	35.7	29.7
Medical social services	2,255	52.8	40.4	12.4
Home health aide/homemaker	4,036	94.5	84.4	10.1
Interns and residents	32	0.8	0.5	0.3
Nutritional guidance	1,016	23.8	17.8	6.0
Pharmaceutical service	272	6.4	3.5	2.9
Appliances and equipment	983	23.0	11.6	11.4

* Data on services provided were missing for 13 of the HHA's operating in January, 1984.

** Data from the Health Care Financing Administration, Providers of Service File.

Source: Williams J., Gaumer G. Cella M. Home health services: an industry in transition, ABT Associates Inc., Washington, D.C. Prospective Payment Demonstration Contract No. 500-84-0021 HCFA. Prepared for the Health Care Financing Administration, May 3, 1984.

Table 8-12. Distribution of persons served, by type of home health service, selected years, 1974-1980.

	1974	1975	1978	1980	Annual compound rate of growth
All persons	392.7	588.7	769.7	957.4	16.0
Nursing care	375.2	564.5	735.9	909.1	15.9
Home health aide	96.0	180.2	261.4	346.6	23.9
Physical therapy	75.3	126.0	178.3	243.3	21.6
Other *	26.1	67.0	95.9	135.4	31.6

Percentage of persons served

	1974	1975	1978	1980	
All persons	100.0	100.0	100.0	100.0	
Nursing care	95.5	95.9	95.6	95.0	
Home health aide	24.4	30.6	34.0	36.2	
Physical therapy	19.2	21.4	23.2	25.4	
Other *	6.6	11.4	12.5	14.1	

* Includes speech or occupational therapy, medical social services and other health disciplines.

Source: Williams, J., Gaumer, G., and Cella, M. Home health services: an industry in transition. ABT Associates Inc., Washington, D.C. Prospective Payment Demonstration Contract No. 500-84-0021 HCFA. Prepared for the Health Care Financing Administration, May 3, 1984.

Table 8-13. Average number of full-time equivalent staff employed by home health agencies, by staff skill level and by auspices, January 1982.*

Type of agency

Staff skill level	Proprietary	Private non-profit	Government	Combined govt. and voluntary	Other non-profit	Other	All agencies
Registered nurse	4.4	3.4	6.6	8.3	10.7	7.6	7.1
Licensed practical nurse	1.6	0.7	0.4	0.8	0.9	0.8	0.9
Physical therapist	1.0	0.9	0.6	1.0	2.0	1.3	1.1
Occupational therapist	0.4	0.3	0.1	0.3	0.6	0.4	0.4
Speech pathologist/ audiologist	0.7	0.4	0.3	0.3	0.8	0.7	0.6
Home health aides	5.2	4.4	2.6	3.1	7.0	4.5	4.8
Others	2.7	3.2	2.6	3.8	7.7	4.4	4.3
Total staff	15.9	13.3	13.2	17.6	29.6	19.7	19.2

* Data from the Health Care Financing Administration, Providers of Service File.

Source: Williams J., Gaumer G., Cella M. Home health services: an industry in transition. ABT Associates Inc., Washington, D.C. Prospective Payment Demonstration Contract No. 500-84-0021 HCFA. Prepared for the Health Care Financing Administration, May 3, 1984.

Table 8-14. Medicare home health services for the elderly: persons served and visits, by age, 1977 and 1980*.

Year & age	Number of enrollees*	Users		Visits		
		Number	Per 1,000 enrollees	Number	Per user	Per 1,000 enrollees
1980						
Total	25,515	888.2	34.8	20,621	23.2	808
65 – 66	3,572	48.3	13.5	1,084	22.4	303
67 – 68	3,335	59.1	17.7	1,324	22.4	397
69 – 70	3,050	66.1	21.7	1,515	22.9	497
71 – 72	2,798	72.6	25.9	1,665	22.9	595
73 – 74	2,459	77.3	31.4	1,789	23.1	727
75 – 79	4,809	203.1	42.2	4,758	23.4	989
80 – 84	3,081	183.5	59.6	4,261	23.2	1,383
85 & over	2,410	178.1	73.9	4,226	23.7	1,753
1977						
Total	23,838	642.9	27.0	14,332	22.3	601
65 – 66	3,349	36.9	11.0	782	21.2	234
67 – 68	3,150	44.2	14.0	976	22.1	310
69 – 70	2,932	49.6	16.9	1,079	21.8	368
71 – 72	2,585	54.0	20.9	1,202	22.3	465
73 – 74	2,310	57.2	24.8	1,267	22.2	548
75 – 79	4,463	146.1	32.7	3,284	22.5	736
80 – 84	2,963	134.4	45.4	3,004	22.4	1,014
85 & over	2,086	117.1	56.1	2,681	22.9	1,285

*Counts of aged persons enrolled in the hospital insurance and/or supplementary medical insurance programs as of July 1.

Note: Based on a 40 percent sample of enrollees.

Source: Waldo D.R., Lazenby H.C. Demographic characteristics and health care use and expenditures by the aged in the United States: 1977–1984. Health Care Financing Review 6: 1: 1–29, 1984.

Table 8-15. Medicaid home health services: payments and recipients and percentage change, 1972-1983.

Year	Vendor payments		Recipients	
	Amount (In millions)	Percentage change	Number (In thousands)	Percentage change
1972	24	-	105	-
1973	25	4.2	110	4.8
1974	31	24.0	144	30.9
1975	70	125.8	343	138.2
1976	134	91.4	319	-7.0
1977	180	34.3	371	16.3
1978	210	16.7	376	1.3
1979	263	25.2	359	-4.5
1980	332	26.2	392	9.2
1981	428	28.9	402	2.6
1982	496	15.9	377	-6.0
1983	596	20.4	422	11.9

Source: Health Care Financing Administration, Office of Financial and Actuarial Analysis, Division of Medical Cost Estimates, 1984.

Utilization increases with age. The greatest increase in the number of users and the number of users per 1,000 enrollees was among those aged 85 and over. They also received a higher average number of visits and a higher number of visits per 1,000 enrollees, both in 1977 and in 1980. The number of users aged 85 and over increased by 52 percent during this three-year period.

Medicaid: Home Health Services

For the United States as a whole, Medicaid home health care reimbursements in 1983 accounted for only 1.85 percent of total Medicaid expenditures. Although Medicaid vendor payments for home health services increased substantially between 1972 and 1983, as shown in Table 8-15, the rate of increase has fluctuated considerably and the overall increase has been considerably less than under the Medicare program. The number of Medicaid home health recipients has also fluctuated, with a net decline in some years. In 1983 the number of recipients was only 23 percent greater than in 1975.

Table 8-16 shows total Medicaid payments, home health payments, and home health payments as a percentage of the total by state in 1983. Home health payments varied by state from less than 0.01 percent in Iowa and Oklahoma to 7.33 percent in New York. Total New York Medicaid expenditures account for 19 percent of all Medicaid expenditures

Table 8-16. Medicaid: total payments and medical vendor payments for home health services, and as a percentage of total Medicaid payments, by state, 1983.

	Total payments	Home health payments	Home health payments as a percentage of total payments
	Numbers in thousands		
United States	32,350,546	597,195	1.85
Alabama	368,732	2,845	0.77
Alaska	51,247	11	0.02
Arizona			
Arkansas	313,208	1,852	0.59
California	3,557,151	4,437	0.12
Colorado	255,305	3,355	1.31
Connecticut	495,413	4,722	0.95
Delaware	62,085	827	1.33
District of Columbia	196,544	4,084	2.08
Florida	681,264	5,920	0.87
Georgia	601,436	8,176	1.36
Hawaii	141,690	437	0.31
Idaho	67,258	221	0.33
Illinois	1,347,004	2,587	0.19
Indiana	596,028	1,961	0.33
Iowa	312,042	2	0.00
Kansas	254,478	726	0.29
Kentucky	410,999	6,933	1.69
Louisiana	674,703	1,306	0.19
Maine	205,072	3,112	1.52
Maryland	446,636	4,778	1.07
Massachusetts	1,338,237	16,692	1.25
Michigan	1,421,703	4,738	0.33
Minnesota	868,114	4,358	0.50
Mississippi	299,391	1,577	0.53
Missouri	468,458	1,373	0.29
Montana	86,170	261	0.30
Nebraska	145,962	1,210	0.83
Nevada	73,706	519	0.70
New Hampshire	93,100	436	0.47
New Jersey	981,531	15,320	1.56
New Mexico	101,780	729	0.72
New York	6,259,549	458,836	7.33
North Carolina	566,993	2,897	0.51
North Dakota	83,319	704	0.84
Ohio	1,474,340	1,672	0.11
Oklahoma	388,659	8	0.00
Oregon	236,231	287	0.12
Pennsylvania	1,718,810	3,134	0.18
Rhode Island	221,733	420	0.19
South Carolina	278,834	1,509	0.54
South Dakota	77,792	495	0.64
Tennessee	508,566	3,620	0.71
Texas	1,316,685	1,427	0.11
Utah	114,519	280	0.24
Vermont	84,272	1,494	1.77
Virginia	488,159	3,170	0.65
Washington	427,142	2,961	0.69
West Virginia	140,626	425	0.30
Wisconsin	901,104	6,681	0.74
Wyoming	24,445	52	0.21

Source: Health Care Financing Administration: Office of Financial and Actuarial Analysis; Division of Medical Cost Estimates, Medicaid Statistics Branch, unpublished data, 1984.

compared with 11 percent for California, and for a massive 77 percent of all Medicaid home health expenditures compared with 0.7 percent for California. The state with the second-highest payments for Medicaid home health services in 1983 was Massachusetts, with 2.8 percent of the total. Whereas an average of 2 percent of all Medicaid recipients received home health services in 1983, 9 percent of the New York Medicaid population received home health care, followed by 3.6 percent of eligible recipients in Massachusetts and Minnesota (see Table 8-17).

Both New York and Massachusetts have introduced prospective payment for Medicaid home health services in an attempt to restrain expenditures.[4]

Medicaid Home Health Expenditures for the Elderly

National data are not available on the characteristics of Medicaid home health care recipients or on the services provided. Of the estimated $8,951 billion in Medicaid long-term care expenditures for the elderly in 1983, 3.2 percent was spent on home health care, representing 63.3 percent of all home health expenditures.[7]

Private Insurance

Many states have recently enacted laws that either require health insurance companies to provide home health care benefits or to offer such coverage to policyholders. In 1984 the number of states with such laws was sixteen.[4] No data are available, however, on the characteristics of the recipients of home health care, on total reimbursements for home health care, or on the proportion of all private health insurance expenditures being paid for home care.

Summary

The Medicare home health care benefit covers a restricted range of home care services related to acute episodes of illness. Although prior hospitalization is no longer required, eligibility for the benefit is determined by the need for "skilled nursing" or rehabilitation services provided to the "homebound." At this time, there is no limit on the number of covered visits, nor are there copayments by the beneficiaries. The benefit is not designed to provide long-term personal and supportive care in the home.

Home health care is also provided under Medicaid, with less restrictive regulations on the scope of service provision than under Medicare. On the other hand, Medicaid expenditures for home health care and the number of recipients have grown at a more modest rate than under the Medicare program for a number of reasons: Medicaid is the payor of last resort, after Medicare and private insurance; reimbursement rates to agencies are lower than under Medicare; and individual states have discretion in determining eligibility for services. It is estimated that nearly 65 percent of Medicaid home health expenditures are for the elderly, a

Table 8-17. Medicaid: total recipients, home health recipients and home health recipients as a percentage of the total, by state, 1983.

	All Medicaid recipients	Home health recipients	Percentage of all recipients
United States	21,494,240	421,798	2.0
Alabama	311,348	3,387	1.1
Alaska	20,038	19	0.1
Arizona			
Arkansas	190,279	2,277	1.2
California	3,499,920	15,900	0.5
Colorado	147,644	3,627	2.5
Connecticut	215,512	4,072	1.9
Delaware	45,618	690	1.5
District of Columbia	117,715	2,066	1.8
Florida	555,213	*58,966	*10.6
Georgia	441,114	7,321	1.7
Hawaii	100,293	461	0.5
Idaho	39,215	327	0.8
Illinois	1,050,992	5,016	0.5
Indiana	271,677	1,890	0.7
Iowa	189,462	2,718	1.4
Kansas	147,201	1,756	1.2
Kentucky	388,041	7,984	2.1
Louisiana	377,957	2,126	0.6
Maine	122,154	2,594	2.1
Maryland	328,012	3,401	1.0
Massachusetts	579,079	20,832	3.6
Michigan	1,187,612	6,787	0.6
Minnesota	326,355	11,760	3.6
Mississippi	290,483	2,491	0.9
Missouri	341,614	2,233	0.7
Montana	44,763	538	1.2
Nebraska	83,963	1,165	1.4
Nevada	27,872	330	1.2
New Hampshire	41,722	1,143	2.7
New Jersey	611,923	6,963	1.1
New Mexico	84,420	859	1.0
New York	2,160,591	194,512	9.0
North Carolina	349,053	3,194	0.9
North Dakota	31,925	593	1.9
Ohio	910,570	6,028	0.7
Oklahoma	232,512	99	0.0
Oregon	153,810	534	0.3
Pennsylvania	1,167,222	10,043	0.9
Rhode Island	104,645	1,418	1.4
South Carolina	236,220	1,979	0.8
South Dakota	33,498	499	1.5
Tennessee	341,243	4,835	1.4
Texas	680,129	2,014	0.3
Utah	66,038	254	0.4
Vermont	53,624	1,030	1.9
Virginia	306,395	2,318	0.8
Washington	257,648	2,763	1.1
West Virginia	177,351	536	0.3
Wisconsin	480,096	6,345	1.3
Wyoming	14,201	35	0.2

*Total Medicaid payments for home health services in Florida do not indicate a high number of recipients, so this is probably a reporting error.

Source: Health Care Financing Administration: Office of Financial and Actuarial Analysis, Division of Medical Cost Estimates, Medicaid Statistics Branch, unpublished data, 1984.

high proprotion of which is for long-term care. Over 75 percent of all federal Medicaid expenditures for home health care is paid to one state—New York.

No national data are available on agencies serving only those who pay privately for home care, but Medicare is a major source of funding for home health care, and the benefit determines the size and operation of a large sector of the home care "industry." Since the liberalization of the benefit in 1981, there has been major growth and change in the number of home health agencies and the number of persons served, with the Medicare home health benefit being the fastest-growing sector of the total Medicare budget. The number of proprietary agencies has grown by about 200 percent, and there have been major increases in the number of institutional-based home care agencies. These trends have been reinforced by the introduction of the prospective payment system for Medicare hospital admissions and the consequent earlier discharge of patients to the community. Means are now being sought to restrain Medicare expenditures for home health care.

Although Medicare reimbursements represent the major income source for certified agencies, most home care agencies also provide services reimbursed by Medicaid or private insurance or paid for out of pocket by the patient. Additional contracts may be made by individual agencies for the provision of services funded under Title III, Title XX, and other sources (see Chapters 9 and 11).

REFERENCES

1. Palmer, H. C. Home care. In Vogel R. J. and Palmer H. C. (eds), Long-Term Care: Perspectives from Research and Demonstrations. Health Care Financing Administration, U.S. Government Printing Office, 1983.
2. Mundinger, M. O'N. Home Care Controversy: too little, too late, too costly. Aspen Books, Rockville, Md. and London, 1983.
3. Cohen, J. Public programs financing long-term care. In Vol. IV, Project to Analyze Existing Long-Term Care Data, The Urban Institute, Washington, D.C., 1983.
4. Williams J., Gaumer G., Cella M. Home health services: an industry in transition. ABT Associates Inc., Washington, D.C. Prospective Payment Demonstration Contract No. 500-84-0021 HCFA. Prepared for the Health Care Financing Administration, May 3, 1984.
5. Home Health Line 9: 71, March 18, 1985.
6. Building a long-term care policy: home care data and implications. Report of the Subcommittee on Health and Long-Term Care of the Select Committee on Aging, House of Representatives. Comm. Pub. No. 98-484, December 1984.
7. Office of Financial and Actuarial Analysis, Health Care Financing Administration, (personal communication).

9

Community and
Social Support Services

Funding for community and social support programs providing services in the home, in adult day care centers, and in other facilities is made available from a variety of sources, including Medicaid and the Social Services Block Grant (Titles XIX and XX of the Social Security Act), Title III of the Older Americans Act, general revenue sharing between the federal and state governments, and state revenues for aging services. In addition, institutional care in nonmedical facilities may be financed by individual states through supplementary payments under the Supplemental Security Income program.

It has been argued that the opportunity for states to "shuffle" funding from overlapping programs is an advantage in maintaining services for beneficiaries, particularly at a time of major reductions in federal public expenditures.[1] On the other hand, the many separate programs involve high administrative costs, and the network of federal and state agencies may create barriers to the development of comprehensive services. Recent federal waivers and initiatives by individual states indicate a growing awareness of the inadequacies and inefficiencies of the present system (see Chapter 11).

Little or nothing is known about nonmedical home-and community-based services because there are no standards for licensing or approving the providers. Data relating to service provision, expenditures, eligibility and client characteristics, either nationally or by state, are unavailable or extremely limited. Legislative and regulatory changes for a number of federally subsidized programs, with differences in funding mechanisms and greater autonomy for the states during the past five years, have meant that less data are available than in the past and that they are not now comparable over time.

The Social Security Act: Title XX

Title XX of the Social Security Act has served as the primary source of federal funding for social services since it was implemented in 1975.

Grants are made to each state to finance the provision of services to needy individuals who meet state-established eligibility criteria.

The program goals established under Title XX include preventing or reducing inappropriate institutionalization by providing for community-based care or other forms of less intensive care; securing referral or admission for institutional care when other forms of care are not appropriate; and achieving or maintaining economic self-support to prevent, reduce, or eliminate dependency.

Until 1982, Title XX provided a closed-ended matching grant: funds were distributed to each state with a ceiling according to population size. The federal government matched each state dollar spent with three dollars of federal money; in return for federal funds, each state was required to meet eligibility, service, and operating requirements. Total federal spending was limited to $3 billion in fiscal year 1981.[2]

Title XX was changed to a block grant under the Omnibus Budget Reconciliation Act of 1981, and the appropriation was reduced to $2.4 billion for 1982. At the same time, federal program requirements were substantially reduced and states were given more flexibility in their use of Title XX funds.[2]

States are no longer required to provide specific services, use a prescribed percentage of federal Title XX funds for services to welfare recipients, or limit the provision of services to families with incomes below 115 percent of the median income of the state. The only federal eligibility requirement remaining is that services must be provided in accordance with the program's original goals.

State reporting requirements were also reduced, but they are still required to develop and make public an annual pre-expenditure report, detailing the types of activities to be funded and the characteristics of individuals to be served. These reports are collected and presented in summary form by the Office of Human Development Services of the DHHS.[3]

In general, the states continue to provide the same services under the block grant as under the previous formula grant program. The most frequently offered services are for home care (homemaker, chore aide, and home management), child day care, and protective and emergency services for children and adults.[3] It was estimated for 1981 that approximately 21 percent of all Title XX program funds benefited the elderly. In 1982 45 states responded to a survey of Title XX administrators and indicated that the majority spent between 10 and 20 percent for services to older persons, with a range from 4.5 to 40 percent. Some states did not maintain age-specific data.[4]

For 1984, the federal Social Services Block Grant authorization was $2.7 billion, a sum less than the Title XX appropriation for 1981. Table 9-1 shows the distribution of proposed services to be provided under Title XX in 1984 by the number of states providing such services. This

Table 9-1. Title XX, Social Services Block Grant: services to be provided by states, 1984*

All services	Number of states
Day-care children	48
Home-based services	47
Protective & emergency services: children	44
Protective & emergency services: adults	42
Adoption	37
Disabled services	34
Foster-care children	34
Information and referral	33
Employment, education & training	30
Family planning services	31
Social support services:	28
Day-care adults	28
Counseling	28
Prevention & intervention	28
Residential care & treatment	26
Transportation services	25
Home delivered/congregate meals	24
Special child & youth services	23
Health related services	23
Foster care adults	20
Legal services	16
Substance abuse services	14
Placement services	13
Housing services	12
Services for unmarried parents	10
Other	27

*Includes 50 States and the District of Columbia.

Source: Social Services Block Grant Pre-ExpenditureReports, Fiscal Year 1984. Office of Human Development Services, Office of Policy and Legislation, Washington, D.C., May 1984.

indicates that home-based services were to be funded from Title XX funds in 47 states.

Title XX funding provides programs for all age groups, eligibility being determined by the individual states or by local agencies, so that in some cases services are available to different categories of recipients according to where they reside within the state. Most states indicate that they make some services available to SSI recipients, and the majority also provide services, such as information and referral without regard to income. Twenty-six states indicated that they impose fees for some services.[3]

Table 9-2 shows the distribution, by state, of selected services that might benefit the elderly. In addition to the 47 states providing home-based services under Title XX, 28 proposed to provide adult day care, 33 information and referral services, and 24 home-delivered and congregate meals.

The fact that a state has not chosen to use Title XX funds for any one of these services does not necessarily imply that they are not available to the elderly, since they may be funded from other sources, either federal or local, and developed by Area and State Agencies on Aging, established under the Older Americans Act for the development and coordination of plans for aging services.[4]

The Older Americans Act: Title III

The Older Americans Act of 1965 provides funding for a variety of services related to home-and community-based care under Title III of the Act (Grants for State and Community Programs on Aging). These include home-delivered and congregate meals; transportation, outreach, information, and referral services; homemaker and home health aide; protective and day care services; residential repair and renovation; and nursing home ombudsmen. In addition, Title III provides funding for the establishment of "multipurpose senior centers" to deliver social and nutrition services and for the organization of recreational and group activities.

The Administration on Aging is the federal agency that was set up to oversee the operation of Older Americans Act programs. In order to receive OAA grants, each state is required to designate one agency to oversee all activities related to the act. State agencies then designate area agencies to oversee planning and service areas, based on factors such as the distribution of the elderly and the need for services within geographic areas. At this writing, there are 57 State Units on Aging and 672 Area Agencies on Aging (AAA's).[5]

AAA's are responsible for planning and coordinating the delivery of social and nutrition services within the planning and service areas. The law requires each area agency to submit an area plan to the state agency for approval, with the ultimate aim of bringing about the development of "comprehensive and coordinated service systems to serve older individuals," using resources efficiently and with a minimum of duplication. This statement of objectives was changed under the 1984 OAA Amendments, (PL98-459) to include the need for "a comprehensive array of community-based, long-term care services adequate to appropriately sustain older people in their communities and in their homes."

AAA's are required to coordinate the administration of their plans with resources available from other federal, state, and local programs for the elderly, including Title XX and other revenues. But previous research has shown that there is little collaboration between Title XX agencies and Area and State Agencies on Aging, and that interagency agreements for the exchange of plans and needs assessment did not guarantee implementation.[4]

Services that may be provided using Title III money come under three headings:

1. Supportive services, including information and referral; transportation; services to assist older individuals to obtain adequate hous-

Table 9-2. Title XX, Social Services Block Grant: distribution of proposed services that may benefit the elderly, by state, 1984.

State	Day care/adults	Disabled services	Foster care/adult	Home-based services	Home delivered/congregate meals	Information and referral	Transport services
Alabama	*	*	*	*	*	*	*
Alaska				*			*
Arizona	*	*		*			*
Arkansas		*	*	*	*	*	
California		*	*	*		*	
Colorado				*		*	
Connecticut	*	*	*	*	*	*	
Delaware	*	*		*	*	*	*
Dist. of Col.	*	*		*		*	*
Florida	*		*	*	*	*	
Georgia	*			*			
Hawaii							
Idaho		*		*	*	*	
Illinois		*		*	*	*	
Indiana	*	*		*			
Iowa	*	*		*			*
Kansas				*			
Kentucky	*	*	*	*	*	*	*
Louisiana		*		*			*
Maine				*	*		*
Maryland	*	*	*	*		*	
Massachusetts				*		*	
Michigan				*		*	
Minnesota				*	*	*	*
Mississippi				*	*		*

Missouri	*			*	*	*	*
Montana	*	*	*	*		*	*
Nebraska	*	*	*	*			*
Nevada				*			
New Hampshire	*	*	*	*	*	*	*
New Jersey	*	*		*	*	*	*
New Mexico				*	*	*	*
New York	*	*	*	*	*	*	
North Carolina	*	*	*	*		*	
North Dakota	*	*	*	*	*	*	*
Ohio				*		*	
Oklahoma	*			*	*		*
Oregon							*
Pennsylvania	*	*	*	*	*	*	
Rhode Island				*	*	*	*
South Carolina	*	*		*		*	
South Dakota	*			*			
Tennessee	*	*	*	*	*	*	
Texas	*	*	*	*	*	*	*
Utah	*	*	*	*	*	*	
Vermont	*	*		*			
Virginia	*	*		*	*	*	*
Washington	*			*	*		*
West Virginia	*		*	*	*	*	
Wisconsin	*		*	*	*		
Wyoming				*			
Total:	28	34	20	47	24	33	25

1. Home-based services include: homemaker, chore aide and home health aide.

Source: Office of Human Development Services, Office of Policy and Legislation.

ing, including residential repair; services designed to assist in the avoidance of institutionalization such as home health services, homemaker, shopping, and escort services; health screening to detect or prevent illness; ombudsman services at the state level for nursing home residents; and services designed for the unique needs of the disabled elderly.
2. Congregate nutrition programs including transportation as well as the actual meals.
3. Home-delivered meals.[2]

AAA's are required to contract with or make grants to providers for the delivery of services rather than providing them directly, unless there is no alternative, as it is argued that the planning and coordination activities of the AAA's might be hindered if they were competing with existing services. Similarly, state agencies are restricted from direct service provision; their main functions are to develop funding formulas for giving money to area agencies and to monitor their administration.

The amount of Title III funds allotted to each state is based primarily on the percentage of elderly in the population. Each state receives four separate Title III allotments: one for state agency administration, one for social services, including those provided by senior centers, one for congregate nutrition services, and one for home-delivered meals.

Several provisions regulate how federal Title III funds are spent. Federal funds may not be used to finance the entire cost of providing services. Each state is required to match its federal social and nutrition service funds with a minimum of 15 percent of its total Title III service costs, at least 25 percent of which has to come from state or local public sources. The remaining nonfederal share of expenditures may be either cash or in kind and may come from public or private funding. A minimum of 25 percent of state and area agency administrative costs must also be financed with nonfederal matching funds.

Although allotments are made separately for each service component of Title III—supportive services and senior centers, congregate and home-delivered meals—there is some transferability between accounts. Up to 20 percent of the total social and nutrition service funds appropriated for any fiscal year may be shifted between nutrition and supportive services "for use as the state considers appropriate."

In addition to federal, state, and local funding, Title III nutrition projects are allowed to accept payments from meal recipients who can afford to pay, and the U.S. Department of Agriculture assists nutrition service providers by donating, through the state agencies, surplus agricultural products.

Eligibility for OAA Title III services is based primarily on being aged 60 or over, but area agencies are required to give preference in the delivery of services to those with the greatest economic or social need, although means testing may not be used to assure preference is given to these individuals.

It is not known what percentage of Title III funds goes to in-home care but, beginning in 1985, AAA's are required to file annual reports specifying how much they spend on three priority areas: access, which comprises transportation, outreach, information, and referral services; in-home services, including homemaker, home health aide, chore aide, visiting, and telephone reassurance; and legal services.

Before 1983 each state was required to provide information on expenditures by service category to the Administration on Aging. Data on OAA Title III expenditures are no longer collected, but a sample survey of AAA's is carried out by the National Association of Area Agencies on Aging (NAAAA). This relates to services being provided and coordinated from all funding sources (Title III, Title XX, state revenues, etc), but there are no comprehensive comparative data by state.[5]

Table 9-3 shows aggregate expenditures by service category for the last two years in which such data were reported to the Administration on Aging, 1981 and 1982. Sixty-six percent of total expenditures under Title III in 1981 were from federal funding, compared with only 62 percent of a higher total in 1982. More than 40 percent of all expenditures in both years were for congregate meals, with a further 11 to 12 percent for home-delivered meals. Access services provided the next major expenditure category, followed by community legal and other services. In-home services accounted for only 7 percent of expenditures.

A similar expenditure pattern is shown in Table 9-4, compiled from the NAAAA Data Base for 1982 and 1983, which includes funding of services from all sources. Again, nearly 40 percent of expenditures were for congregate meals in 1983, with a further 13 percent for home-delivered meals. Housekeeping, chore service, and repairs and renovations amounted to only 7 percent of the total.

A survey of AAA's conducted since the introduction of prospective payment for hospital care under Medicare shows a major increase in referrals of elderly persons to AAA's for the provision of in-home services, including case management, home nursing, housekeeping, and personal care services. These referrals are for care not reimbursed under the Medicare home health benefit.[6]

Area Agency on Aging: Client Characteristics

There are no national data on client characteristics and utilization of services developed by Area Agencies on Aging. The development of a client services information center has, however, been funded by the District of Columbia Office on Aging to monitor services provided to the elderly, for reimbursement purposes, for client tracking, and for management reporting.[7] The population is not characteristic of the elderly pop-

Table 9-3.   Older Americans Act: Title 111 expenditures by service category and percentage distribution, fiscal years 1981 and 1982.

	Fiscal year 1981		Fiscal year 1982	
	(Expenditures in thousands)			
	Amount	Percentage	Amount	Percentage
Total outlays (Federal and non-federal)	$898,489	100.0	$931,141	100.0
Total Federal	595,604	66.0	578,981	62.0
Area plan Administration:	56,271	6.3	57,484	6.2
Supporting services:				
Access	140,075	15.6	144,856	15.6
In-home	627,780	7.0	62,155	6.7
Community (legal)	19,475	2.2	19,231	2.1
Community (all other)	95,627	10.6	102,032	11.0
Services in care facilities	2,093	0.2	6,199	0.7
Senior center facilities	23,587	2.6	14,980	1.6
Nursing home Ombudsman	5,418	0.6	6,594	0.7
Congregate meals:				
Meals	305,892	34.0	311,209	33.0
Project management	71,040	7.9	81,669	8.7
Supporting services	16,190	1.8	12,803	1.4
Home delivered meals:				
Meals	72,317	8.0	77,329	8.3
Project management	13,872	1.5	17,724	1.9
Delivery costs	10,710	1.2	14,105	1.5
Supporting services	3,142	0.3	2,742	0.3

Source: Department of Health and Human Services: Administration on Aging, Washington, D.C., unpublished data.

ulation in the country as a whole, but the data are of interest in documenting utilization of community-based support services.

Only 27 percent of the total population of Washington, D.C., is white (174,705 of 638,333) compared with 70 percent black (448,370 of 638,333) and 3 percent of other races. The black population is predominantly young, however, and for older age groups the proportion of blacks and whites is more comparable. Among those aged 75 and over there are

Table 9-4. National Data Base on Aging: Area Agency on Aging service expenditures, 1982 and 1983.***

Service activity	Percentage of expenditures	
	1983*	1982**
Meals - congregate	38.48	35.33
Meals - home delivered	13.23	11.08
Transportation	9.41	10.14
Income support/material aid	4.48	4.48
Information	3.76	6.01
Housekeeping	3.37	6.09
Recreation	3.15	6.16
Counseling	2.36	1.98
Client finding (outreach)	2.16	1.76
Advocacy (includes legal)	2.14	1.83
Chore service	2.13	3.09
Repairs/maintenance/renovations	1.96	0.84
Personal care	1.93	2.49
Assessment (client)	1.76	1.76
Referral	1.54	1.74
Placement	1.40	2.44
Instruction/training	1.32	1.97
Visiting	1.02	0.50
Escort service	0.90	0.45
Supervision	0.59	1.28
Physical fitness	0.54	0.14
Telephoning	0.54	0.41
Evaluation	0.41	0.43
Shopping	0.39	0.23
Treatment (medical)	0.27	0.35
Diagnosis (medical)	0.22	0.18
Discount	0.20	0.26
Guardianship	0.19	0.17
Letter writing/reading	0.11	0.05
Interpreting/translating	0.04	0.02

* Total = $161,429,600 from 111 Area Agencies on Aging.

** Total = $263,054,269 from 151 Area Agencies on Aging

*** Based on all Area Agency on Aging funding sources, including the Older Americans Act Title III.

Source: National Data Base on Aging: services for older persons. Supported by State and Area Agencies on Aging. National Association of Area Agencies on Aging, Washington, D.C., July 1983.

almost equal numbers of blacks and whites (13,766 whites and 13,947 blacks).[8]

While there are many missing values for most services in the District of Columbia Office on Aging data, particularly for counseling, congregate meals, and recreational and social activities, the data do provide insight

Table 9-5. Area Agency on Aging: number of clients and percentage distribution by
age and service category, October 1, 1983 - September 30, 1984.

| | Age group | | | | | | |
	Under 65	65-74	75-84	85-94	95 & over	Missing data	Clients served
Service				Number			
All services	1,894	4,337	3,047	903	124	8,246	18,551
Assessment	24	78	104	55	12	98	371
Case management	41	151	197	101	20	260	770
Congregate meals	920	2,235	1,410	296	40	2,119	7,020
Counseling	989	2,312	1,609	473	68	2,983	8,434
Day care	33	113	95	22	6	49	318
Home meals	203	498	520	191	32	757	2,201
Home health	43	97	110	60	6	45	361
Homemaker	3	27	47	36	5	259	377
Legal	208	293	183	44	9	1,342	2,079
Recreational/social	816	2,174	1,339	274	30	2,101	6,734
Transport of meals	85	229	297	110	15	533	1,269
Escort transportation	141	244	230	67	11	170	863
Transportation	289	794	477	95	10	851	2,516
Weekend meals	84	211	144	19	0	715	1,173
				Percentage			
All services	18.4	42.0	29.6	8.7	1.3	44.5	100.0
Assessment	0.1	0.3	0.4	0.2	0.0	26.4	100.0
Case management	8.0	29.6	38.7	19.8	3.9	33.8	100.0
Congregate meals	18.8	45.6	28.7	6.0	0.8	30.2	100.0
Counseling	18.1	42.4	29.5	8.7	1.3	35.4	100.0
Day care	12.3	42.0	35.3	8.2	2.2	15.4	100.0
Home meals	14.1	34.5	36.0	13.3	2.3	34.4	100.0
Home health	13.6	30.7	34.8	19.0	1.9	12.5	100.0
Homemaker	2.5	22.9	39.8	30.5	4.2	68.7	100.0
Legal	28.2	39.8	24.8	6.0	1.2	64.6	100.0
Recreational/social	17.6	46.9	28.9	6.0	0.6	31.2	100.0
Transport of meals	11.5	31.1	40.3	15.0	2.1	42.0	100.0
Escort transportation	20.3	35.2	33.1	9.7	1.5	19.7	100.0
Transportation	17.4	47.7	28.7	5.7	0.6	33.8	100.0
Weekend meals	18.3	46.1	31.4	4.1	0.0	61.0	100.0

Source: Georgetown University, Department of Community and Family Medicine,
Client Services Information System. Project funded by the District of Columbia
Office on Aging, Washington, D.C.

into the characteristics of individuals with high utilization of social and
community support services by service category.

A disproportionate number of those aged 75 and over received case
management, home-delivered meals, home health care, and homemaker
services (see Table 9-5). Seventy-two percent of clients were female com-

Table 9-6. Area Agency on Aging: number of clients and percentage distribution by sex and service category, October 1, 1983 - September 30, 1984.

Service	Male	Female	Missing data	Clients served
		Number		
All services	3,403	8,660	6,488	18,551
Assessment	3	230	68	371
Case management	139	435	196	770
Congregate meals	1,493	3,600	1,927	7,020
Counseling	1,685	4,133	2,616	8,434
Day care	110	168	40	318
Home meals	459	1,075	667	2,201
Home health	115	206	40	361
Homemaker	84	208	85	377
Legal	392	1,368	319	2,079
Recreational/social	1,318	3,492	1,924	6,734
Transport of meals	228	561	480	1,269
Escort transportation	222	507	134	863
Transportation	422	1,291	803	2,516
Weekend meals	171	306	696	1,173
		Percentage		
All services	28.2	71.8	35.0	100.0
Assessment	24.1	75.9	18.3	100.0
Case management	24.2	75.8	25.5	100.0
Congregate meals	29.3	70.7	27.5	100.0
Counseling	29.0	71.0	31.0	100.0
Day care	39.6	60.4	12.6	100.0
Home meals	29.9	70.1	30.3	100.0
Home health	35.8	64.2	11.1	100.0
Homemaker	28.8	71.2	22.5	100.0
Legal	22.3	77.7	15.3	100.0
Recreational/social	27.4	72.6	28.6	100.0
Transport of meals	28.9	71.1	37.8	100.0
Escort transportation	30.5	69.5	15.5	100.0
Transportation	24.6	75.4	31.9	100.0
Weekend meals	35.8	64.2	59.3	100.0

Source: Georgetown University, Department of Community and Family Medicine, Client Services Information System. Project funded by the District of Columbia Office on Aging, Washington, D.C.

pared with 28 percent male (see Table 9-6). Men were more likely to receive day care, home health care, and weekend meal services; a disproportionate number of women received case assessment, case management, and transportation services.

Of all those receiving services, only 23 percent were married, compared with 53 percent who were widowed and a further 25 percent who were divorced, separated, or never married (see Table 9-7). As might be predicted, the highest use of services was by those living alone—over 50 percent of all clients. Twenty percent of services were used by those living

Table 9-7. Area Agency on Aging: number of clients and percentage distribution by marital status and service category, October 1, 1983 - September 30, 1984.

Marital status

	Never married	Married	Widowed	Separated	Divorced	Missing data	Clients served
				Number			
All services	1,229	2,525	5,882	773	783	7,359	18,551
Assessment	8	71	143	12	12	105	371
Case management	67	112	268	23	28	272	770
Congregate meals	620	1,064	2,451	394	378	2,113	7,020
Counseling	610	1,240	2,808	384	387	3,005	8,434
Day care	62	40	114	25	23	54	318
Home meals	134	347	809	81	72	758	2,201
Home health	33	108	143	11	13	53	361
Homemaker	4	15	24	1	5	328	377
Legal	143	282	1,100	117	115	322	2,079
Recreational/social	535	1,048	2,322	328	360	2,141	6,734
Transport of meals	73	178	428	30	28	532	1,269
Escort transportation	104	139	314	46	49	211	863
Transportation	196	339	883	125	134	839	2,516
Weekend meals	71	83	215	52	44	708	1,173
				Percentage			
All services	11.0	22.6	52.6	6.9	7.0	39.7	100.0
Assessment	10.5	26.7	53.8	4.5	4.5	28.3	100.0
Case management	13.5	22.5	53.8	4.6	5.6	35.3	100.0
Congregate meals	12.6	21.7	49.9	8.0	7.7	30.1	100.0
Counseling	11.2	22.8	51.7	7.1	7.1	35.6	100.0
Day care	23.5	15.2	43.2	9.5	8.7	17.0	100.0
Home meals	9.3	24.0	56.1	5.6	5.0	34.4	100.0
Home health	10.7	35.1	46.4	3.6	4.2	14.7	100.0
Homemaker	8.2	30.6	49.0	2.0	10.2	87.0	100.0
Legal	8.1	16.1	62.6	6.7	6.5	15.5	100.0
Recreational/social	11.6	22.8	50.6	7.1	7.8	31.8	100.0
Transport of meals	9.9	24.2	58.1	4.1	3.8	41.9	100.0
Escort transportation	16.0	21.3	48.2	7.1	7.5	24.4	100.0
Transportation	11.7	20.2	52.7	7.5	8.0	33.3	100.0
Weekend meals	15.3	17.8	46.2	11.2	9.5	60.4	100.0

Source: Georgetown University, Department of Community and Family Medicine, Client Services Information System. Project funded by the District of Columbia Office on Aging, Washington, D.C.

with a spouse; the highest proportion was for home health care. For those living with a child, adult day care was the most frequent service used (see Table 9-8).

Additional data show that 85 percent of clients were nonwhite, 18 percent received SSI payments, and a high proportion received food stamps and rent subsidies. These data reflect the income differentials between the elderly black and white populations of the District of Columbia and indicate the role played by community and social support services in assisting

Table 9-8. Area Agency on Aging: number of clients and percentage distribution by living arrangement and service category, October 1, 1983 - September 30, 1984.

	Alone	With spouse	With child	With relative	Other	Missing data	Clients served
				Living arrangements			
				Number			
All services	5,804	2,217	1,137	958	968	7,467	18,551
Assessment	40	61	16	30	25	99	371
Case Management	275	90	37	66	48	254	770
Congregate meals	2,345	915	500	394	546	2,320	7,020
Counseling	2,647	1,114	638	525	514	2,996	8,434
Day care	45	39	50	41	97	46	318
Home meals	758	326	112	137	88	780	2,201
Home health	94	96	51	41	24	55	361
Homemaker	20	14	4	9	3	327	377
Legal	1,216	219	144	104	113	283	2,079
Recreational/social	2,248	903	441	333	455	2,354	6,734
Transport of meals	339	171	82	99	46	532	1,269
Escort transportation	227	131	101	79	123	202	863
Transportation	743	288	213	161	206	905	2,516
Weekend meals	288	75	34	25	30	721	1,173
				Percentage			
All services	52.4	20.0	10.3	8.6	8.8	40.3	100.0
Assessment	51.5	22.4	5.9	11.0	9.2	26.7	100.0
Case management	53.3	17.4	7.2	12.8	9.3	33.0	100.0
Congregate meals	49.9	19.5	10.6	8.4	11.6	33.0	100.0
Counseling	48.7	20.5	11.7	9.7	9.5	35.5	100.0
Day care	16.5	14.3	18.4	15.1	35.6	14.5	100.0
Home meals	53.3	22.9	7.9	9.6	6.2	35.4	100.0
Home health	30.7	31.4	16.7	13.4	7.9	15.2	100.0
Homemaker	40.0	28.0	8.0	18.0	6.0	86.7	100.0
Legal	67.7	12.2	8.0	5.8	6.3	13.6	100.0
Recreational/social	51.3	20.6	10.1	7.6	10.4	35.0	100.0
Transport of meals	46.0	23.2	11.1	13.4	6.3	41.9	100.0
Escort transportation	34.3	19.8	15.3	12.0	18.6	23.4	100.0
Transportation	46.1	17.9	13.2	10.0	12.8	36.0	100.0
Weekend meals	63.7	16.6	7.5	5.5	6.6	61.5	100.0

Source: Georgetown University, Department of Community and Family Medicine, Client Services Information System. Project funded by the District of Columbia Office on Aging, Washington, D.C.

the low-income elderly with coordination and provision of nutrition, home management, and other supportive services.

Medicaid

Personal Care Option

In addition to federal funding of in-home services under Title XX and the Older Americans Act, states may provide an optional class of services under Medicaid, identified in federal regulations as "personal care services in a recipient's home." This allows nonagency and nonprofessional providers, other than members of the recipient's family, to deliver services that are prescribed by a physician and supervised by a nurse. Personal care services may include assistance with personal hygiene, dressing, eating, and ambulation, but some states cover homemaker, case management, and habilitation services under "personal care," even though they are not mentioned in the Medicaid statute.[2]

In 1980 eighteen states offered personal care services under their Medicaid programs, but the majority avoided coverage of nonmedical services and have preferred to finance in-home and community care services through their own programs or Title XX rather than risk creating an expensive entitlement under Medicaid (see Table 9-9).[1]

Personal care expenditures in fiscal year 1980 totaled $217 million, which was over 50 percent more than the $141 million spent for home health care under Medicaid. New York accounted for almost 90 percent of the total spending, followed by Oklahoma with $17 million and Texas with $4 million. In these states Medicaid expenditures for personal care were substantially higher than for home health care.[2]

Adult Day Care

Another service provided under Medicaid in some states is adult day care. This encompasses a range of maintenance, rehabilitative, and social programs to assist elderly and disabled persons living in the community. Such programs may provide a variety of medical, personal care, and social services to impaired individuals who are unable to live entirely independently but who may be maintained in the community with this supportive care.

Adult day care is not specifically identified in Medicaid regulations but is funded under regulations relating to "preventive, diagnostic, therapeutic, rehabilitative or palliative services, provided to an outpatient by, or under the direction of, a physician."[2]

Apart from Medicaid, adult day care programs are also made available under funding from Title XX and the Older Americans Act, while Medicare will cover utilization of certain specified services for eligible recipients, regardless of site, if they are prescribed by a physician.

In 1980 there were 617 adult day care programs in 46 states developed under the three sources of federal funds.[9] As shown in Table 9-9, only eight states used Medicaid funding.

For information on services provided under the Medicaid Home and Community-Based Long-Term Care Waiver Program (Section 2176), see Chapter 11.

Supplemental Security Income (SSI)

SSI is widely used to finance nonmedical institutional care through state supplementation programs. Established in 1974 to provide a national

Table 9-9. Medicaid non-institutional long-term care: states providing personal care and adult day care, 1981.

State	Personal care	Adult day care
Alabama		
Alaska		
Arizona		
Arkansas	*	
California		*
Colorado		
Connecticut		
Delaware		
District of Columbia	*	
Florida		
Georgia	*	*
Hawaii		
Idaho		
Illinois		
Indiana		
Iowa		
Kansas	*	*
Kentucky		
Louisiana		
Maine		
Maryland	*	*
Massachusetts	*	*
Michigan	*	
Minnesota	*	
Mississippi		
Missouri		
Montana	*	
Nebraska	*	
Nevada	*	
New Hampshire	*	
New Jersey		*
New Mexico		
New York	*	*
North Carolina		
North Dakota		
Ohio		
Oklahoma	*	
Oregon	*	
Pennsylvania		
Rhode Island		
South Carolina		
South Dakota	*	
Tennessee		
Texas	*	
Utah		
Vermont		
Virginia		
Washington		*
West Virginia		
Wisconsin	*	
Wyoming		

Source: Cohen J. Public programs financing long-term care, in Vol. IV, Project to Analyze Existing Long-Term Care Data. The Urban Institute, Washington, D.C., 1983.

minimum income for the aged, blind, and disabled poor, SSI regulations allow states to establish minimum income levels above the federal standards through supplemental payments that are not counted as income in calculating federal benefits, (see Chapter 3). By the end of fiscal year 1980, 33 states had established optional supplementation programs for eligible individuals residing in nonmedical facilities or receiving some type of home-based personal care.

The living arrangements chosen for supplementation by the states range from basic foster care in homes or small group settings to larger institutions providing both personal care and continuous supervision. Most states that offer supplements for long-term care restrict them to recipients living in nonmedical institutions—domiciliary care facilities, personal care homes, homes for the aged—which provide varying amounts of personal assistance.[3] States relying on SSI to finance board and care homes may use Medicaid home health or personal care funds to finance nursing, home health aide, and other supportive services for residents.[1] Thus there is some substitution of SSI payments, which are largely federally financed, to individuals for board and care at lower cost to the state than if care were provided in intermediate care facilities under the Medicaid program.

Table 9-10 shows the number of recipients, federal and state expenditures, and average monthly payment to those with nonmedical long-term living arrangements in states that have opted for administration of the program by the Social Security Administration.[2] Seventy percent of the recipients and 75 percent of the expenditures for these 15 states were accounted for by California and New York.

For nonmedical facility residential care, it was estimated that in fiscal year 1980, 73.1 percent was financed by SSI compared with 4.0 percent under Title XX and 22.9 percent by the Veterans Administration.[2]

Summary

Community and social support services, assisting the elderly to remain in their homes and avoid institutional care, are provided from a variety of federal funding sources including the Social Services Block Grant, Medicaid, and Title III of the Older Americans Act, together with general revenue sharing between federal and state governments and state revenues for aging services. (There is additional funding and direct provision of services through churches and other charitable organizations.)

Services may range from home-delivered meals and assistance with personal hygiene to legal services and adult day care. Some services, such as those developed from Title XX funds, are made available to eligible individuals of all ages; other services, including those funded under Title III and state revenues for aging services, are developed specifically for the elderly. Many states do not choose to take advantage of all the federal

Table 9-10.   Federal and state expenditures on optional state supplements to recipients living in non-medical long-term care facilities, for states with federally administered Supplemental Security Income programs, 1982*

	Recipients	Federal & state expenditures (In thousands)	State expenditures (In thousands)	Average state monthly payment
Total	126,017	494,124	294,468	194.74
California	59,748	246,036	147,792	206.13
Delaware	343	1,020	420	103.28
District of Columbia	746	2,125	1,344	149.60
Hawaii	1,570	5,544	3,048	161.78
Iowa	95	240	60	49.62
Maine	2,552	6,804	2,712	88.50
Massachusetts	4,174	13,980	8,052	160.73
Michigan	17,899	63,480	34,176	159.13
Montana	703	2,136	696	82.74
Nevada	245	660	492	170.29
New Jersey	4,704	15,036	7,176	127.19
New York	28,637	120,000	80,488	234.10
Pennsylvania	1,265	4,260	2,052	135.35
Vermont	1,422	4,176	1,788	104.85
Wisconsin	1,914	7,680	4,212	183.41

*Unpublished data from the Social Security Administration, Office of Research and Statistics.

Source: Cohen J., Public programs financing long-term care, in Vol. IV, Project to Analyze Existing Long-Term Care Data.   The Urban Institute, Washington, D.C., 1983.

funding available, particularly under the Medicaid program, in order to avoid creating an expensive entitlement for care. Some states supplement federal SSI payments to provide housing in nonmedical board and care homes, with additional assistance from community and social support services, for individuals who might otherwise be institutionalized at greater expense to the state under the Medicaid program.

In recent years states have been given greater freedom in the use of funds under some of these programs; at the same time, federal reporting requirements have been reduced. As a result, less national data are now available than in the past on the distribution of funds between services and on the characteristics of those receiving services. There are therefore no indicators for assessing the adequacy of service provision or coverage. Nor are there data on agencies providing services under the various forms of community and social service funding because there are no standards for licensing providers. Agencies may, however, be subject to state or local regulation.

Available information does indicate that there is considerable variation both within and between states in total social and community service financing available, in the administrative framework established for the various funding sources, in the services available, and in eligibility for such services. There may be overlapping and duplication in some areas and gaps in service provision in others. In one state an individual may receive assistance with personal hygiene from a personal care aide employed directly by a state Medicaid agency, homemaker services from a proprietary agency with a contract to provide services with Title XX funding, and meals provided through a nutrition program established with Title III funds. Individuals in other states, or in different areas of the same state, may be less well served.

The area agencies set up under Title III for the development of long-term care services to maintain the elderly in their communities and in their homes are required to coordinate their plans with resources available from other federal, state, and local programs. In the past, there has been little collaboration between the agencies established to administer the various funds, even when there have been coordination agreements.

It has been argued that there are benefits in the variety of funding sources because of the opportunities provided to maintain services when restrictions are imposed on any individual program. On the other hand, the large number of agencies established to provide services under the separate programs results in high administrative costs and in difficulties in obtaining information and access for clients and their families.

Data on the characteristics of clients from one agency on aging show that a high proportion of services are delivered to low-income, elderly women living alone and that adult day care is the most frequently used service for those living with a child and home health care for those with a spouse. Although these services seem to be reaching the appropriate client groups, it is not known how comprehensive they are in serving the overall needs of dependent elderly persons in the community, because there are no outcome measures.

Some recent evidence indicates that earlier discharge of Medicare patients from hospitals under the prospective payment system may result in cost-shifting from the Medicare program to the community and social support services, which are already of doubtful adequacy, for patients discharged from hospitals with limited family or financial assets.

REFERENCES

1. Feder J., Scanlon W. J. Fiscal incentives in federal-state financing for long-term care. In, Vol. IV, Project to Analyze Existing Long-Term Care Data, The Urban Institute, Washington, D.C. 1983.

2. Cohen, J. Public programs financing long-term care. In, Vol. IV, Project to Analyze Existing Long-Term Care Data, The Urban Institute, Washington, D.C., 1983.
3. Social Services Block Grant, Pre-Expenditure Reports, Fiscal Year 1984. Office of Human Development Services, Office of Policy and Legislation, Washington, D.C., May 1984.
4. Developments in aging: A Report of the Special Committee on Aging, U.S. Senate, Washington, D.C. U.S. Government Printing Office, 1983.
5. National Data Base on Aging: services for older persons supported by State and Area Agencies on Aging, 1982. National Association of Area Agencies on Aging, Washington, D.C., July 1983.
6. Harlow K. S., Wilson L. B. DRG's and the Community-Based Long-Term Care System. Presented to the Committee on Education and Labor, Subcommittee on Human Resources, U.S. House of Representatives, July 30, 1985.
7. Georgetown University, Department of Community and Family Medicine, Client Services Information System. Project funded by the District of Columbia, Office on Aging.
8. U.S. Bureau of the Census: General Social and Economic Characteristics, District of Columbia, (PC80-1-C10), 1980 Census of the Population, Washington, D.C. U.S. Government Printing Office, July, 1983.
9. Palmer H. C. Adult day care. In, Vogel R. J. and Palmer H. C. (eds), Long-Term Care: Perspectives from Research and Demonstrations, Health Care Financing Administration, U.S. Government Printing Office, 1983.

10
The Veterans Administration

The Veterans Administration (VA) provides disability compensation and pensions for former military personnel and their survivors and medical and related care for eligible veterans. The VA health care system was established to provide service-disabled veterans with health care for service-related conditions. Approximately 10 percent of the patients fall into this category. An additional 20 percent are service-disabled veterans with conditions unconnected with their actual service activities; special groups including aged and indigent veterans account for the remaining 70 percent of patients treated in VA facilities.[1]

At present, the VA operates a vast network of health facilities and programs that are administered locally by 172 medical centers throughout the country. Long-term care constitutes a large component of VA services, including nursing home care in both VA and private nursing homes, domiciliary care in VA facilities, personal care and supervision in residential care homes, hospital-based home care, aid to state-administered veterans' homes at all levels of care, and a number of other benefits that help aged and disabled veterans to avoid institutional care.[1]

Over the next twenty years there will be a major change in the age structure of the veteran population, and the VA will have to address the issue of rapidly increasing demands on their health care system. Assuming that there are no further wars in this century, the total number of veterans will decline, but the average age will increase significantly. Seventy-five percent of the 11.1 million veterans who served in World War II will reach age 65 by 1990, so that the number of veterans aged 65 and over will more than double between 1985 and 1995. By 2000, the 9 million veterans aged 65 and over will represent 37 percent of the veteran population; by 2015, 45 percent of the veteran population will be aged 65 and over. Between 1980 and 2000 there will also be 136-percent increase in the number of veterans aged 85 and over.[2]

The cost of VA health care for the aged in the future will rise due to the increasing numbers of elderly veterans and the higher per capita cost of providing health care for the aged.

Eligibility for VA Services

VA medical benefits are available to all veterans who have service-connected disabilities and to all those aged 65 and over who have nonservice-connected disabilities. Other veterans with nonservice-connected disabilities may be eligible for hospital and nursing home care, depending on availability and income.

Total potential demand for VA care is dependent on the number of those who are aware of and actively using VA services, the number who are eligible but not aware of VA provisions, and the number who are eligible and aware but do not choose to use their benefits.

At present, many eligible veterans do not seek VA health services, and having private insurance lowers the probability of use. Veterans using the VA system in 1977 were more likely to be poor, elderly, have less education, and suffer from service-connected disabilities.[3] There is high utilization by younger veterans with psychiatric disorders.

Long-Term and Extended Care Provision

Nursing Homes

The VA owns and operates nursing home care units in 45 states, providing skilled nursing care and related medical services to eligible veterans. This is the largest and most costly long-term care program in the VA system.

In addition to this program, the VA pays for skilled or intermediate level care for veterans in private nursing homes under the Community Nursing Home Care Program. Every VA medical center operates such a program, contracting nationwide with a total of nearly 3,000 homes. The VA determines a maximum number of approved placements across the country that may be operating on a given day, and an allotment is made to each medical center.

Each center negotiates its own reimbursement rates, subject to a national maximum. Nearly all placements in community nursing homes are for patients following discharge from a VA acute hospital stay or from a VA domiciliary. Patients with service-connected disabilities may receive care at VA expense indefinitely; those with nonservice-connected disabilities are limited to six-months coverage.

Domiciliaries

The VA operates domiciliary care facilities in 15 states. These provide medical and other care to ambulatory veterans who are disabled by age or injury but who do not require acute hospital or skilled nursing care. Eligibility for the program depends on chronic disability and inability to earn a living, but with income limitations. The domiciliary care program serves primarily a younger population of whom 55 percent in 1978 had a psychiatric disorder as a primary diagnosis.

The program has shifted from primarily custodial care to the provision of therapeutic, preventive, and rehabilitation care. Some patients are placed in a domiciliary care facility following acute hospital or nursing home care, with the intention of returning them to the community within a year; others are admitted for long-term custodial care.[1]

State Veterans Home Program

The VA system of nursing and domiciliary care homes is supplemented by a system of state homes that provide nursing and domiciliary care for veterans. Individual states are responsible for the establishment and administration of these homes, and the VA gives financial assistance through two different grant programs. Under one program the VA may pay the state up to 65 percent of the cost of constructing, expanding, and altering approved facilities; under the other the VA pays a subsidy for each veteran on a per diem basis, up to a maximum number of authorized beds. The state-operated facilities are also permitted to charge veterans for the cost of their care, collecting from their pensions and other income.

Eligibility and admission requirements are determined by the individual homes. Most homes require that prospective patients be disabled by disease or age and unable to support themselves. Some require active wartime service, and almost all require state residency of two to five years. Some admit only male veterans; others admit wives and widows of veterans who meet other eligibility requirements.

Community Residential Care

This program provides room, board, and limited personal supervision to veterans who do not need hospital or nursing home care. The VA inspects private homes and provides patient placement, supervision, and follow-up services, even though the home is selected by the individual veteran. The veteran pays for his care in the home, usually with VA-provided funds from pensions or compensation payments.[1,2]

In June 1981 118 VA centers had residential home care programs, placing a total of 13,500 patients. Seventy-one percent of these patients had a psychiatric disorder as the primary diagnosis, and 32 percent were aged 65 and over.[1]

Hospital-Based Home Care

Hospital-based home care programs were started in 1970. The programs are staffed and administered by VA personnel and are designed to provide medical, nursing, social, dietetic, and rehabilitative services in the homes of nonambulatory or housebound patients. The range of services provided includes drugs, supplies, equipment, and diagnostic tests as well as direct nursing care and ongoing assessment and planning for meeting the patient's social, psychological, rehabilitation, and nutrition needs. Homemaker and housekeeping services are not included.

Eligibility criteria include the physician's assessment that the patient does not require inpatient care but does need professional care, the absence of which would result in hospitalization. The home environment must be one in which daily care can be provided by family members or others who agree to the proposed plan of care.

Home care is provided for up to twelve months after acute hospital care and is terminated when the condition that resulted in the patient's enrollment is deemed stable. The physician has the discretion to extend the period of treatment. At the time of termination, the VA social worker is responsible for making community referrals.[1]

A rural home care program is also being developed to evaluate the efficiency and determine the costs of serving a target population of medically isolated patients.[2]

Adult Day Health Care

This provides medical, rehabilitation, social, recreational, and health education services to veterans in a congregate setting during normal working hours. These are usually, but not exclusively, elderly veterans in need of supportive and rehabilitative care to maintain functioning and enable them to stay in their own homes. (These are distinguished from VA day hospitals and day treatment centers, which are primarily directed to the adjustment of the younger, psychiatrically disabled veteran.)[2]

Other VA Programs for Long-Term Care

In addition to cash payments under disability compensation and pension programs, the following provisions form part of the extended care system, helping aged and disabled eligible veterans to remain in their homes or in the community:

> *The aid and attendance program* provides additional disability compensation or pension benefits to veterans who are housebound or in need of regular aid and attendance of another person because of their disabilities.
>
> *The automobile or other conveyances program* provides a one-time payment toward the purchase of a vehicle to veterans with certain impairments of mobility and/or vision.

The clothing allowance provides an annual stipend to the service-connected disabled veteran when prosthetic or orthopedic devices tend to damage clothing.

The prosthetic appliances program pays for prosthetic aids for eligible veterans.

The specially adapted homes program provides grant money up to 50 percent of the cost of buying, building, or remodeling a home specially adapted to the needs of certain permanently and totally disabled veterans.[1]

DATA SOURCES

Sources of information for the tables presented in this chapter are as follows:

The Veterans Administration publishes an annual report, and additional data are provided in other publications from the Office of Reports and Statistics.[2,4] VA data are also reported by the Health Care Financing Administration in the context of total national health care expenditures.[5,6]

Demographic Changes

In the absence of future wars, the veteran population is projected to show a progressive decline of nearly 50 percent between 1980 and 2030, from 29 to 15 million (see Table 10-1). The population aged 65 and over, however, will increase from 3 to nearly 9 million between 1980 and 2000, accounting for 37 percent of the total veteran population in 2000 compared with 11 percent in 1980. The veteran population aged 75 and over is projected to show an increase of nearly 450 percent between 1980 and 2000[2] and, for those aged 85 and over, the projected increase between 1980 and 2010 is from 216,000 to 1.4 million.

VA Institutional Care

Table 10-2 shows the average number of beds, average daily census, and number of patients treated in VA-funded institutions. There are nearly 80,000 beds in acute care hospitals, and a further daily average of 23,000 patients were being cared for in VA-funded nursing home facilities plus 16,000 in domiciliary care programs.

In addition, there are 30 hospital-based home care teams in operation and another 30 planned by 1990. In 1983 approximately 168,000 home visits were made and 7,400 patients were treated.[2]

Utilization and Expenditures

The total VA budget in 1983 was $24.9 billion, and 31 percent of total expenditures ($7.6 billion) was for medical care. Eighty-three percent of

Table 10-1. Veterans population by age cohort, selected years, 1980-2030.*

Year	Total Veterans population	Aged Veterans			
		Total 65 & over	65-74	75-84	85 & over
		(Numbers in thousands)			
1980	28,640	3,036	2,177	643	216
1982	28,522	3,506	2,753	450	303
1985	28,014	4,833	3,792	778	262
1990	27,064	7,155	5,621	1,326	208
1995	25,802	8,516	5,846	2,359	311
2000	24,259	8,974	5,007	3,451	516
2010	20,710	8,125	3,723	3,020	1,383
2020	17,461	7,771	4,053	2,351	1,367
2030	15,086	5,716	2,065	2,476	1,175
		Percentage of all Veterans			
1980		10.6	7.6	2.2	0.8
1982		12.3	9.7	1.6	1.1
1985		17.3	13.5	2.8	0.9
1990		26.4	20.8	4.9	0.8
1995		33.0	22.7	9.1	1.2
2000		37.0	20.6	14.2	2.1
2010		39.2	18.0	14.6	6.7
2020		44.5	23.2	13.5	7.8
2030		37.9	13.7	16.4	7.8

*Data from the Veterans Administration Office of Reports and Statistics.

Source: Veterans Administration: Caring for the Older Veteran. U.S. Government Printing Office, Washington, D.C., July 1984.

all medical expenditures were made to provide care in 172 VA medical centers and other hospitals.

Nearly 28.2 million individuals were eligible to receive medical benefits in 1983. VA medical centers provided care for 1.3 million inpatients, and 18.5 million outpatient visits were made. Over 24 million inpatient days of care were financed by the Veterans Administration in VA and non-VA hospitals. An additional 9.5 million inpatient days were provided in VA nursing homes or financed by the VA in state- or community-operated nursing facilities.[5]

VA Care for the Elderly

Although elderly veterans make up only 12.3 percent of the total veteran population, they accounted for 27 percent of all hospital discharges and 32.1 percent of all medical and surgical discharges in 1982. The length of stay for elderly veterans averaged 31.9 days compared to 26.6 days for all veterans.[6] As shown in Tables 10-3 and 10-4, there is a disproportionately

Table 10-2. Veterans Administration: inpatient care summary, 1982.

Facility	Average operating beds	Average daily census	Admissions	Discharges and deaths	Patients treated	Total	Short term (99 days or less)	
							Days	Percent of total discharges
Hospital care:								
VA medical centers	79,859	64,992	1,216,348	1,217,123	1,280,468			
Total hospital care		66,634	1,249,690	1,250,621	1,315,244			
Extended care:								
Nursing home care								
VA medical centers	9,414	8,849	7,520	7,213	16,473	392.6	27.5	52.0
Community nursing homes		10,212	23,923	23,529	34,092	145.3	41.8	47.1
State home nursing *a/*b	9,198	6,919	5,687	4,836	12,228			
Total nursing home care		25,980	37,130	35,578	62,793			
Domiciliary care:								
VA Medical centers & domiciliary	8,201	6,852	6,378	7,050	14,067	441.3	39.2	48.8
State home domiciliaries *a/*b	7,661	4,489	4,468	4,579	8,914			
Total domiciliary care	15,862	11,341	10,846	11,629	22,981			
Total extended care		37,321	47,976	47,207	85,774			
Total inpatient care		103,955	1,297,666	1,297,828	1,401,018			

*a Operating beds not reported.

*b Average length of stay not available for state home facilities.

Source: Summary of Medical Programs, Veterans Administration Office of Reports and Statistics, September 1983.

Table 10-3. Percentage use of Veterans Administration institutional care, by age, 1982.

Age	Percentage of users	Hospitals			Domiciliaries		Nursing homes		
		General	Psychiatric	State	VA	State	VA	State	Community
Under 45	14.9	19	29.8	1	9	3	2.7	1.0	4.2
45–54	14.1	6	18.8	8	19	14	7.3	4.6	8.2
55–64	33.9	36	31.8	26	44	41	27.7	23.1	30.3
65–74	20.6	19	14.8	23	22	25	25.9	26.6	27.8
75–84	8.1	6	5.6	18	5	11	16.0	17.5	13.6
85 & over	8.4	5	4.2	25	2	6	20.5	27.1	15.9

Source: Veterans Administration Patient Treatment File, Office of Reports and Statistics, 1982.

Table 10-4. Use of Veterans Administration hospital and nursing home care by aged veterans: 1982

Age	Veterans Population (March 1982) (In thousands)	Hospital patients discharged from VA facilities		Nursing home patients discharged from VA and community facilities			
		Number	Rate per 1,000 Veterans	VA nursing home care units	Community nursing home care units	Total	Rate per 1,000 Veterans
Total	28,522	956,881	33.5	5,773	17,826	23,599	0.8
65 & over	3,506	258,482	73.7	3,545	11,037	14,582	4.2
65-74	2,753	175,600	63.8	1,511	4,973	6,484	2.4
75-84	450	44,901	99.8	850	2,720	3,570	7.9
85 & over	303	37,981	125.4	1,184	3,344	4,528	14.9

Source: Veterans' Administration Annual Report, 1982. U.S. Government Printing Office, Washington, D.C., 1982.

high utilization by elderly veterans of all institutional services in relation to their numbers in the elderly population. Table 10-4 shows the number and rate per 1,000 veterans, by age, using hospital and nursing home care. The discharge rate per 1,000 veterans aged 65 and over is four times that of the total veteran population. Utilization by the population aged 85 and over is highest, with 14.9 discharges per 1,000 veterans.[6]

Summary

The VA provides a more comprehensive range of acute and long-term care services and related cash grants to eligible veterans than is available to other sectors of the population. Most of the services are given at no cost to the beneficiary, but access may be limited by local availability. There are, for instance, a limited number of home care programs.

The effectiveness and efficiency of the services provided may be open to question. Average length of acute hospital stay is considerably longer in VA than in other acute hospitals. The uptake of services by eligible veterans is low, and there is little use by those with alternative forms of health insurance. Given the known characteristics of those with high use of the present system, restrictions on VA provision would undoubtedly increase the demand for care under local Medicaid programs.

It is difficult to predict the future demand for VA services as a result of a major increase in the number of elderly veterans. Based on present utilization by veterans living in the community, it was recently estimated that if the number of elderly veterans doubled, the increase in service use would be about 16 percent.[3] This would undoubtedly be higher as a result of any restriction on the present Medicare benefit.

Furthermore, the potential utilization of VA long-term care services is unknown. The holding of private insurance lowers use of the VA system, but private insurance and Medicare coverage for nursing home and home care services is minimal. The projected growth in the number of veterans of advanced old age could therefore lead to a significant increase in the demand for long-term care services provided or funded by the VA.

REFERENCES

1. Cohen J. Public programs financing long-term care. In, Vol. IV, Project to Analyze Existing Long-Term Care Data, The Urban Institute, Washington D.C., July 1983.
2. Veterans Administration: Caring for the Older Veteran. Office of Reports & Statistics, Washington, D.C., U.S. Government Printing Office, July 1984.
3. Horgan, C., Taylor A., Wilensky G. Aging veterans: will they overwhelm the VA medical care system? Health Affairs 2: 3: 77–86, 1983.

4. Veterans Administration: veteran population projections by age and period of
   service, selected years 1984–2030. Office of Reports & Statistics, Statistical
   Policy & Research Service, Washington, D.C., U.S. Government Printing
   Office, April, 1983.
5. Gibson R. M., Levit, K. R., Lazenby H., Waldo D. R. National health expenditures, 1983. Health Care Financing Review, 6: 2: 1–29, 1984.
6. Waldo D. R., Lazenby H. C. Demographic characteristics and health care use
   and expenditures by the aged in the United States: 1977–1984. Health Care
   Financing Review 6: 1: 1–29, 1984.

11

Research, Demonstrations, and Initiatives in Long-Term Care

Recognition of the constantly increasing need for long-term care services in the aging population, a growing awareness of the inadequacies of present programs in terms of service coverage and administrative fragmentation, and pressure to restrain the constantly increasing costs of the total health care system are all factors contributing to the search for cost-effective alternatives in provision and funding of long-term care. There have been several recent federal and state initiatives to reform the present system. Large- and small-scale research and demonstration projects for both institutional and community care services have been funded. Projects relating to long-term care have also received substantial funding from private institutions such as the Robert Wood Johnson Foundation.

Federal Programs

Federal funding for research and demonstration projects comes from a number of agencies, including the Administration on Aging (AOA) under Title IV of the Older Americans Act, the National Center for Health Services Research (NCHSR), and the Health Care Financing Administration (HCFA). Title IV funds have been awarded to develop multidisciplinary long-term care and gerontology centers in universities and research institutions nationwide. Model projects relating to primary care, the provision of medical social services to the homebound, and other areas of care for the noninstitutionalized elderly have been funded by the AOA. Title IV funds may be used to cover research and demonstration program costs for up to three years, but not to pay for direct services reimbursable under Medicare, Medicaid, or Title XX.[1]

Congress has passed legislation authorizing waivers to the Medicare and Medicaid regulations for research, demonstrations, and innovation in the provision and reimbursement of long-term care services. As a result, waivers have been granted to allow both state and federal agencies to adopt certain initiatives or to undertake research and demonstration projects with regard to both nursing home and community care. Waivers for projects relating to the Medicare program may be granted under Section 222 of the Social Security Act and for Medicaid under Section 1115 of the 1972 amendments to the Social Security Act.

In addition, Section 2176 of the Omnibus Budget Reconciliation Act of 1981 authorized the granting of waivers to state Medicaid agencies to offer home and community-based services to recipients as an alternative to institutionalization.

Federally funded research and demonstration programs tend to focus on: alternatives to institutional long-term care, the population that is best served by these alternatives and the cost of provision, or alternative reimbursement strategies that offer incentives for long-term care providers to be efficient in delivering services and responsive to the needs of long-term care patients.[2]

State Programs

State initiatives with regard to long-term care include: funding individual research and demonstration projects, with or without additional federal grants; applying for federal waivers to implement new long-term care programs; adopting alternative reimbursement methods for Medicaid providers; and using the state taxation system to assist the elderly living in the community and to provide incentives to families and individuals for assuming greater responsibility in the provision of long-term care.[3]

In many instances, state Medicaid agencies wish to change coverage, procedures, or reimbursement in an attempt to achieve certain objectives. In general, the Health Care Financing Administration encourages states to experiment with their present Medicaid programs, particularly where the results may benefit other state programs.[2]

Research and Demonstration Projects

Research and demonstration projects involving federal and/or state funding, together with federal program waivers, have been carried out for introducing and evaluating changes in the provision of both institutional and community care.

Nursing Homes

Medicare waivers were granted in 1977 to Blue Cross and Blue Shield of Oregon and Massachusetts to conduct demonstrations in eliminating the three-day prior hospitalization requirement for skilled nursing facility coverage.[2] Legislation was passed in 1982 to eliminate the prior hospitalization requirement, but has not been implemented (see Chapter 6).

Both Wisconsin in 1978 and New York in 1980 were awarded Section 1115 waivers to test methods for improving the quality of care in nursing homes. The Wisconsin study sought to reallocate the time of nursing home surveyors to those facilities cited as having deficiencies and away from those known for the provision of good care. The New York study made use of a screening survey developed for the Wisconsin project.[2]

Community Care

Projects that have sought to carry out client assessments and provide appropriate, integrated community care as an alternative to institution-alization include the following:

In 1974 Connecticut initiated the Triage model, based on a single entry access point to the health delivery system for the elderly Medicare pop-ulation, using state funding, a grant from the Administration on Aging, funding from the National Center for Health Services Research, and Sec-tion 222 Medicare waivers.[2,4]

The New York State legislature established the Long-Term Home Health Care (ACCESS) Program in 1978, offering an alternative to insti-tutionalization for Medicaid clients meeting the medical criteria for nurs-ing home care. In this instance the New York State Department of Social Services received Medicaid waivers under Section 1115 of the Social Security Act to assist in the three-year demonstration program.[2,5]

The Wisconsin Community Care Organization and Georgia Alterna-tive Health Services projects have also used a combination of federal waivers and federal and/or state funding for community-based demon-stration projects.[6-7]

These studies have demonstrated success in implementing the provi-sion of coordinated care for elderly persons in the community with out-come measured in increased satisfaction for the recipients. The results have been variable in terms of cost-effectiveness and control.

In 1978 an experimental study of adult day care and homemaker ser-vices was carried out at two sites in New York state, one in San Francisco and one in Lexington, Kentucky, to test the effect on patient outcomes and utilization costs. Although neither of the services is covered under Medicare at present, the costs were reimbursed under a Section 222 waiver.[8,9] This study concluded that adult day care represented a major additional cost to the Medicare program and did not contribute to improved functional status.

None of these studies, whether evaluated as successful or otherwise, has led to major legislative or regulatory changes, but further research initiatives in providing integrated community care services have been funded.

In 1980 fifteen states were given Title IV grants by the AOA to develop plans for the implementation of more effective statewide planning and the coordination and allocation of long-term care resources. These State System Development Grants were awarded to California, Delaware, Illinois, Idaho, Colorado, Washington, Oregon, Minnesota, Rhode Island, Wisconsin, Arkansas, South Dakota, North Carolina, New Hampshire, and the District of Columbia.[1]

Major research and demonstration projects being conducted at the time of writing are the following.

National Long-Term Care Channeling Demonstration Program

The largest discretionary project funded by the AOA, in conjunction with the Health Care Financing Administration and the Office of the Assistant Secretary for Planning and Evaluation (ASPE), is the national channeling demonstration program. Contract awards were made to twelve states to test the extent to which long-term care services can be delivered at home or in the community at the same or lower cost compared with institutions. The program emphasizes client assessment and case management and includes, in addition to the service component, contracts for technical assistance and program evaluation. The design and planning phase of the projects was completed in early 1982. Two variants of channeling were proposed for testing in the demonstration: (1) the basic case management model, superimposing a coordinating and accountability mechanism on the present system of long-term care services; and (2) the financial control model, modifying the first variant to address issues of cost control and strengthen the project's ability to enhance access to needed services.[5]

The states awarded channeling demonstration contracts were Florida, Hawaii, Kentucky, Maine, Maryland, Massachusetts, Missouri, New Jersey, New York, Ohio, Pennsylvania, and Texas. As part of the demonstration program, each is required to establish an interagency long-term care planning group, with members nominated by the governor to prepare a statewide long-term care plan.

Social/Health Maintenance Organization Program for Long-Term Care

In 1980, the Health Care Financing Administration awarded a three-year planning grant to the University Health Policy Consortium at Brandeis University to develop the concept of the Social/Health Maintenance Organization (S/HMO) under the general research and demonstration authority provided by Section 1115 of the Social Security Act.

The aim of the S/HMO is to provide a complete range of social and health maintenance services under a fixed capitation fee through one responsible nonprofit provider organization. This addresses two major problems in the delivery of long-term care: the fragmentation of service delivery systems and of funding sources.

The S/HMO is an approach to the organization of health and social services in which the elderly, including those at high risk of institutionalization, are voluntarily enrolled by a managing provider into an integrated service system. Acute care hospital, nursing home, ambulatory medical care, and personal care support services, including home health, homemaker, and chore services, are to be provided by or through the S/HMO for a fixed, annual, prepaid capitation fee. The S/HMO provider will share the risk for service expenditures and act as broker for other needed services, integrating health and social services under the direct financial management of the provider at the point of service delivery.

In the proposed demonstration the S/HMO will serve persons from a targeted elderly population, ranging from the ambulatory nonimpaired elderly to the severely disabled. Financing will come from the combination of public funding through Medicare, Medicaid, Title XX, and Title III, as well as from private payments, deductibles, and private third-party payments.[2]

HCFA has provided grant support for the development of a comprehensive prepaid service plan for Medicare and Medicaid recipients at one demonstration site in each of the following states: California, Minnesota, New York, and Massachusetts.[2] In addition, Minnesota was awarded a grant by HCFA to test the feasibility of providing all Medicaid benefits, including long-term care services, on a prepaid capitated basis.

It is hoped that these demonstrations will provide information on the development of actuarially sound capitation rates and on the benefits derived from the integration of Medicare and Medicaid coverage by a central care provider.[3]

Prospective Payment for Long-Term Care Services

The 1983 amendments to the Social Security Act changed Medicare reimbursement for acute hospital care from cost-based to prospective payments based on predetermined rates. The introduction of the same system for nursing home care is under consideration, and the Health Care Financing Administration is now funding a major national demonstration program to test the feasibility of introducing prospective payment of the Medicare home health benefit. The demonstration, based on approximately 120 home health agencies, was due to begin in October 1985 but has been delayed.[10]

State Initiatives in Long-Term Care

There has recently been a wide range of state initiatives in the provision and funding of both institutional and community-based long-term care.

State Taxation

A number of state legislatures are using the tax system to promote policies relating to long-term care. Income tax deductions may be allowed for expenses incurred by individuals in caring for an elderly relative in the home. In Idaho tax-deductible voluntary contributions may be made by the relatives of nursing home patients toward the state share of nursing home costs. In Virginia authority was granted to local governing bodies to allow total or partial exemption of the elderly from real estate taxes to help them maintain residence in the community.[3]

Institutional Care

As previously described, some states utilize Supplemental Security Income payments to finance living arrangements in nonmedical institutions such as domiciliary care facilities, personal care homes, and homes for the aged (see Chapter 9).

Many state Medicaid agencies have sought to control costs by introducing prospective payment for nursing home care. Some states have introduced preadmission screening or prior authorization for nursing home admission. Preadmission screening may be used to determine which nursing home applicants might be maintained in the community at lower cost. In Virginia it is now stipulated that Medicaid coverage will not be available to an individual who enters a nursing home as a private pay patient and subsequently spends down to Medicaid eligibility unless the individual has undergone preadmission assessment.[3]

Preadmission screening with a view to substituting community-based for nursing home care would tend to result in admission of only the most severely disabled. If less disabled, lower-cost patients are replaced by those requiring more care, there will be pressure to increase the per diem rates, which already show substantial variation by state.[3]

Some states have anticipated this by introducing other reimbursement methods, including the adoption of patient-specific or case-mix measures to compensate for patients with greater care needs. ADL scores may be used to adjust rates for individual patients. In at least one state higher rates are paid for patients who have been "backed up" in hospitals for prolonged periods awaiting nursing home admission.[3]

Medicaid Eligibility

Changes recently introduced by a number of states could have a major impact on the number of individuals eligible for long-term care and could encourage a shift from institutional to community-based care.

One measure has been to increase the income eligibility standards for individuals residing in the community who need long-term care services to the higher standards allowed for those admitted to nursing homes.

In addition, nursing home coverage is likely to be restricted by the fact that most states have taken advantage of the increased latitude in federal law granted under the Tax Equity and Fiscal Responsibility Act of 1982 to deny Medicaid eligibility to individuals who transferred resources at less than market value in order to obtain Medicaid coverage and to attach a lien on the real property of Medicaid recipients who are permanently institutionalized.[3]

Competitive Bidding

Until 1981, Arizona was the only state not to have introduced a Medicaid program. The Arizona Health Care Cost Containment System, authorized by the Health Care Financing Administration, was introduced as an alternative to traditional Medicaid systems. Among other features, the program has prepaid capitated financing and a competitive bidding process to select the providers who participate in the program.[11] The system has the potential for the development of comprehensive, community-based acute and long-term care with lower rates of hospital and nursing-home use.

Section 2176 Waivers

The Medicaid Home and Community-Based Long-Term Care Waiver Program, Section 2176 of the Omnibus Reconciliation Act, 1981, provides a range of policy options for states with regard to the reallocation of resources from nursing home to community care provision. Section 2176 authorizes the granting of waivers to state Medicaid agencies so that they may offer home- and community-based services to recipients as an alternative to institutionalization, and it addresses some of the biases toward institutional care prevalent within the Medicaid eligibility provisions.

The population groups for whom the program was developed are the aged and disabled, the mentally retarded and developmentally disabled, and the chronically mentally ill.[3] Funding of services is available only for individuals who would otherwise require nursing home placement at the intermediate care facility (ICF) level. States may request a waiver to provide community-based services to persons not receiving SSI cash assistance who have incomes up to 300 percent of the federal payment standard, thus allowing states to provide assistance to individuals who would otherwise not be eligible for Medicaid unless they were institutionalized.

In addition, a separate category of 2176 waivers known as "model" waivers was created to facilitate state efforts to provide community-based services to individuals who are considered to be inappropriately institutionalized as a result of the income eligibility rules of the SSI program. These rules prohibit individuals who are living at home from receiving SSI and, in most instances, Medicaid, because the income and resources of a spouse or parents are considered to be available or "deemed" to the individual. Under the 2176 "model" waivers, individuals may become eligible for care provided under Medicaid while living at home instead of in institutions. Coverage under model waivers is limited nationally to no more than 50 blind and/or disabled children and adults.[12]

Table 11-1 summarizes the ways in which the standard Medicaid regulations are modified under the 2176 waiver program. Two specific Medicaid requirements may be waived: that Medicaid services be available

Table 11-1. Summary of changes to the Medicaid program under 2176 Waivers for Home and Community-Based Care.

Medicaid Requirements	Medicaid Waiver Program
"Statewideness"	
Services covered under a State's plan must be available throughout the State.	Services may be targeted to State-selected geographic areas.
Long-Term Care Services	
Required:	May include a wide range of services: case management, homemaker, home health aide, personal care, adult day care, habilitation, respite, and other services defined by the State and approved by HHS.
* Skilled nursing facility	
* Home health services for persons entitled to skilled nursing facility services.	
Allowed:	
* Intermediate care facility services	
* Personal care, adult day care under certain circumstances.	
Eligibility	
Must meet Medicaid income eligibility requirements, except that higher income levels may apply to persons in institutions.	Expanded to include persons with higher income levels living in the community.
Costs of Services	
No budget ceiling	Home and community-based services for individuals under the waiver must not exceed the cost of care in institutions.

Source: O'Shaughnessy C., Price R. Medicaid 2176 Waivers for Home and Community-Based Care. Congressional Research Service, The Library of Congress, Washington, D.C., June 1985.

throughout a state and that covered services be equal in amount, dura-tion, and scope for certain Medicaid recipients. Although the statute allows states to cover a broad array of services not previously reimburs-able under Medicaid, the administrative implementation limits the pos-sible increase in available community and social support programs. States are constrained from serving more individuals under the 2176 Waiver than they would have done in its absence, and the average per capita Medicaid expenditure may not exceed what it would have been without the waiver. Waivers do not therefore create a statewide entitle-ment to any program and, in many cases, cover only a small number of eligible persons in selected areas.

Services that may be provided under the waiver program are: case management, homemaker, home health aide, personal care, adult day care, habilitation, respite care, and other services requested by Medicaid agencies and approved by the Health Care Financing Administration as cost effective.

As of April 30, 1985, a total of 167 waiver requests had been submitted by 47 states, of which 95 had been approved, 36 were still pending, 14 had been withdrawn, and 22 were disapproved. Of those approved, over 50 percent were targeted to the elderly/disabled. Seventeen were model waivers.[12] Waivers are granted for a period of three years.

Because of the legislative requirement that states provide for an eval-uation of an individual's need for community-based services, the service most frequently offered under the waivers is case management. As shown in Table 11-2, 31 states offer case management to aged/disabled individ-

Table 11-2. Medicaid 2176 Waivers for Home and Community-Based Care: number of states, by service offered and eligibility group, April 1985.*

	Eligibility group		
Service	Aged/ Disabled	Mentally retarded/ Developmentally disabled	Mentally ill
Case management	31	30	2
Homemaker	26	11	-
Home health aide	11	6	-
Personal care	18	9	1
Adult day care	26	14	2
Habilitation	4	31	1
Respite	24	25	2

* Does not include model waivers.

Source: Health   Care   Financing   Administration,   Office   of   Research   and Demonstrations, unpublished data, April 1985.

Table 11-3. Medicaid 2176 Waivers for Home and Community-Based Care: number of approved waivers, by service offered, April 1985.*

Service:	Number of waivers
Case management	66
Homemaker	39
Home health care	16
Personal care	28
Adult day health	43
Habilitation	36
Respite care	52

* Does not include model waivers.

Source: Health Care Financing Administration, Office of Research and Demonstrations, unpublished data, April 1985.

uals and 30 to mentally retarded/developmentally disabled. Table 11-3 indicates that of the 95 programs presently approved, 66 programs (nearly 70 percent) offered case management. The next most popular services for the elderly were homemaker and adult day care, neither of which are reimbursable under Medicare, and have only been made available under Medicaid in a few states by liberal interpretation of the regulations (see Chapter 9).

The Health Care Financing Administration plans to conduct both internal and independently contracted evaluations of the 2176 waiver program to assess its impact. While the diversity of waiver programs makes for interesting experimentation, it makes evaluation of the program's cost-effectiveness more problematic, particularly in discerning which program combinations are more or less effective in achieving cost savings.[13]

REFERENCES

1. Cohen J. Public programs financing long-term care. In, Vol. IV, Project to Analyze Existing Long-Term Care Data, The Urban Institute, Washington, D.C., 1983.
2. Hamm L. V., Kickham T. M., Cutler, D. A. Research, demonstrations and evaluations. In, Vogel R. J. and Palmer H. C. (eds), Long-Term Care: Perspectives from Research and Demonstrations, Health Care Financing Administration, U.S. Government Printing Office, 1983.
3. Staff Data and Materials Related to Medicaid and Long-Term Care. Report to the U.S. Senate, Committee on Finance, November 1983.
4. Hicks B. C., Quinn J. L. Triage: coordinated delivery of services to the elderly. Final Report, Grant No. HS02563 National Center for Health Serv-

ices Research, Office of the Assistant Secretary of Health, DHEW, December 1979.
5. Eggert G. M., Bowlyow J. E., Nichols C. W. Gaining control of the long term care system: first returns from the ACCESS experiment. The Gerontologist 20: 356–363, 1980.
6. Applebaum R., Seidl F. W., Austin C. D. The Wisconsin Community Care Organization: preliminary findings from the Milwaukee experiment. The Gerontologist 20: 350–355, 1980.
7. Skellie F. A., Coan R. E. Community-based long-term care and mortality: preliminary findings of Georgia's alternative health services project. The Gerontologist 20: 372–379, 1980.
8. Palmer H. C. Adult day care. In, Vogel R. J. and Palmer H. C. (eds) Long-Term Care: Perspectives from Research and Demonstrations; Health Care Financing Administration, U.S. Government Printing Office, 1983.
9. Weissert W., Wan T., Livieratos B., Katz S. Effects and costs of day-care services for the chronically ill. Medical Care XVIII: 567–584, 1980.
10. Williams J., Gaumer G., Cella M. Home health services: an industry in transition. ABT Associates Inc., Washington, D.C. Prospective Payment Demonstration Contract No. 500-84-0021 HCFA. Prepared for the Health Care Financing Administration, May 3, 1984.
11. Christianson J B., Hillman D. G., Smith K. R. The Arizona experiment: competitive bidding for indigent medical care. Health Affairs 2: 3: 88–103, 1983.
12. O'Shaughnessy C., Price R., Medicaid 2176 Waivers for Home and Community-Based Care. Congressional Research Service. The Library of Congress, June 1985.
13. Health Care Financing Administration. Short-Term Evaluation of Medicaid: Selected Issues: Grants and Contracts Report, HCFA Pub. No. 03186, Office of Research and Demonstrations, Washington, D.C. U.S. Government Printing Office, 1984

12

International Comparisons of Population Aging and Long-Term Care Financing and Provision

Reduction in mortality rates for older age groups and consequent increases in life expectancy and in the size of the elderly population is not a phenomenon unique to the United States. Most nations, whether industrialized or less developed, are facing major increases in the number of both elderly and very aged individuals.[1] In all societies aging is accompanied by declining income and increasing rates of chronic morbidity and functional disability. As a result of historical, social, political, and economic factors, different countries have developed and implemented different health and social support programs for their elderly and disabled populations. Many programs were introduced when life expectancy was shorter and the elderly represented a much smaller proportion of the population.[2]

In view of the almost universal increase in the elderly population, the growing dependency ratios of older to younger persons, and the rising proportion of national expenditures for care and support of the elderly, it is of interest to compare the experiences of different countries for at least two distinct reasons.

There is considerable cross-national variation in rates of increase in life expectancy at different ages and in age-, sex-, and cause-specific mortality rates. It is therefore of interest to seek associations between declining mortality and health care expenditures, per capita national income, and lifestyle variables to identify the factors having positive or negative effects on mortality rates. This could have important implications for countries with less favorable outcomes.

Additionally, it appears that many countries have provided a greater range of health and social services for a relatively larger elderly population than exists in the United States while expending a lower proportion of gross national product for such programs.[2,3] A comparison of types of provision and funding of health and social services for the elderly could indicate cost-effective alternatives in the delivery of care in the United States.

Data on population growth and life expectancy are available for most countries, but some additional information for comparison with U.S. data on national expenditures and provision of health and other long-term care services have been obtained for Canada, the Scandinavian countries, the Netherlands, France, West Germany, the United Kingdom, and Japan. These countries are of particular interest for a number of reasons.

Japan, with its recent history of industrialization, also has the longest life expectancy in the world for both men and women and is now experiencing a major growth in the proportion of the population aged 65 and over. Western Europe already has a higher proportion of both elderly and very aged individuals than other areas of the world and has a longer history of industrialization and of health and social service provision. For example, the Sickness Insurance Act was introduced in Germany in 1883 and the National Health Insurance Act in Britain in 1911.[4] The United States and Canada are roughly forty years behind Western Europe in the aging of their populations, and Canada probably offers the best foreign comparison with the United States in that it encompasses a large geographic area, has a federal form of government, and has a similar population age distribution.[2,5]

Although standardized international reporting systems provide demographic and mortality data that make possible valid international comparisons over time, there are considerable difficulties in comparing health and social programs between countries because of differences in organization, financing, and definitions of services. It is therefore necessary to have a general understanding of the differences in the funding and provision of health and other long-term care services and the ways in which the definitions of services may vary.

Health Care Financing and Organization

In contrast to the United States, all the Western European countries for which data were obtained, as well as Canada and Japan, provide universal access to health care for their populations. All systems include some national government subsidy and regulation, but the means by which they are financed vary widely from country to country. Examples include the following: Sweden has national health insurance funded from national and local tax revenues, social insurance contributions, and modest copayments by patients for some care; Germany has developed a complicated system of private insurance, provider associations, and sickness funds, providing health care coverage and cash benefits for illness, with capital expenditures financed directly by the government; since 1948 the United Kingdom has had a national health service funded by general tax revenues with copayments for some items such as prescription drugs; Japan has nonprofit, pre-paid, employment-based insurance, with government subsidy to insure universal coverage since 1961, and comprehensive free care for the aged since 1973; Canada adopted a system of national health insurance in the late 1960's, financed partly by the federal government, with contributions by employers and employees, but with each provincial government responsible for implementing its own plan.[2,3,6,7]

The mechanisms for controlling costs all relate to the structure of the individual systems. In the Scandinavian countries most health facilities are publicly owned and operated, and most physicians are salaried employees of the state. In Germany contractual agreements are often made between medical associations and the sickness funds, with statutory fee schedules negotiated for physician services and per diem rates for hospital care for those not entering into fixed contracts. There are similar arrangements in Japan, which also has the lowest hospitalization rates of any of the countries studied—a major factor in controlling costs. In the United Kingdom total health expenditures are limited by government budget authorization, family practitioners are paid a capitation fee per patient, and hospital physicians are salaried employees. In Canada, as in the United States, voluntary hospitals and fee-for-service physicians are the predominant providers of health care, but there are national guidelines and standard formulas for controlling costs, with hospital budgets negotiated by the provinces on a global basis together with fee schedules for physicians.[3,5,8]

In all the countries studied there is a disproportionately high rate of admission of elderly persons to acute hospitals and, although no other system attempts to regulate acute hospital admissions and length of stay by linking eligibility for care to specific, defined acute episodes of illness, as under Medicare in the United States, there is concern with "blocked" beds, and backup by the elderly waiting transfer to long-term facilities in many countries, including Canada, the United Kingdom, and Denmark.[8-11]

Long-Term Care

In all countries long-term care provision consists of both institutional and community care, but the range and definitions of services and their financing and administration vary from country to country. Most health care systems provide a sizable component of long-term care, both institutional and community based, but nonmedical care in the home and residential accommodation for the less impaired is frequently under the aegis of social service departments or housing authorities. In the United Kingdom, for example, the administration of health services, including community nursing, is delegated to district health authorities; social service provision and housing are the responsibility of local government. There are similar divisions in other countries, and the administrative fragmentation and lack of coordination of services are perceived frequently to be a problem.[2,8]

Definitions of institutions for long-term care vary between countries. One cross-national study concluded that although long-term care for the elderly in the United States was thought of almost entirely in terms of nursing home provision, there was no true equivalent in the European countries studied.[8] Canada does, however, have a system of proprietary, voluntary nonprofit, and public institutions that conform to the American model of nursing home care, although there is a smaller for-profit sector than in the United States.[5] In Europe long-term institutions include geriatric and psychogeriatric beds and wards in hospitals and homes for the aged.[2] Residential accommodation and forms of congregate or sheltered housing for the frail and impaired elderly provided outside the health care system are not necessarily categorized as "institutions." Community care includes a wide range of health and social support services that may include home nursing, geriatric visiting, home help/homemaker care, "meals-on-wheels," shopping, night-sitting, laundry service, and home improvements. Day care in geriatric hospitals and rehabilitation and recreational centers and transportation to these facilities is also frequently provided in European countries, as is respite care to relieve the burden of families in caring for the elderly and disabled.[2,8]

In many cases the commitment to long-term care outside institutions for as many impaired elderly as possible is an explicit government policy, notably in the United Kingdom and Scandinavia.[2] In these countries health-related services are usually provided directly by nurses, health visitors, aides, and other staff employed by the local health authorities, who work in close liaison with primary care physicians. Other services such as homemaker and meals-on-wheels are provided by staff employed by social service departments or in cooperation with voluntary associations. Services are usually universally provided (subject to local variations in availability) with charges for domestic help and meals.

In contrast with other European countries, cash benefits instead of services are frequently provided by sickness funds in Germany to enable the elderly to buy needed care. In other countries with high rates of service provision, such as Sweden and the United Kingdom, supplementary cash payments or attendance allowances are often paid the disabled elderly and their caregivers to encourage independent living. In some European countries family members may be paid to provide care to the elderly; a significant proportion of home help aides in Sweden are relatives of elderly persons receiving the service.[2]

European comparisons may be of interest but of limited relevance to the United States because of fundamental differences in political philosophies, administrative structures, and systems of health care delivery and financing. The Canadian experience is of greater significance because of the similarities with the United States. National health insurance was introduced by the Canadian provincial governments between 1968 and 1972; long-term care benefits for nursing home and home care have been added to the insurance coverage at different times and in different forms.[5,7]

Before universal long-term care benefits were introduced, eligibility for nursing home care was on the basis of means-tested benefits, similar to the Medicaid program in the United States. It has been argued that it was the "frustration" of mixing welfare sponsorship for nursing home care with universal coverage for medical care that led the provinces to insure long-term care.[5]

Nursing home care is now insured with no means or asset test; functional impairment is the basis for eligibility. Clients pay a moderate room charge set at a rate to leave all individuals with a small discretionary income. Proprietary agencies are paid on a per diem basis annually negotiated for the whole province, and annual budgets are prospectively negotiated for nonprofit facilities.[5]

Home care is free and, unlike the Medicare benefit in the United States, includes both home health care and homemaker services. Care and assistance are provided subject to assessment of need by a case manager. In some provinces there is direct employment of staff by the government agencies; in others services are provided by a mixture of for-profit and voluntary agencies, particularly for homemaker services.

The Canadian approach to long-term care therefore differs from other universally funded systems in its mix of for-profit and nonprofit providers; the resulting competition is seen as benefiting both the government and the clients.[5] It is clearly a model with the potential for adaptation to the future funding and provision of long-term care in the United States.

DATA SOURCES

Most countries have standardized vital statistics registration systems from which demographic, morbidity, and life expectancy data are regularly aggregated and reported so that valid cross-national comparisons can be made.[12]

For comparisons of health and long-term care financing and utilization, tables have been derived from a range of national and international sources, including the United Nations, the budget and departmental reports of individual governments, and academic papers and publications. It is therefore impossible to assume strict comparability of data due to differences in reporting methods and in definitions of services between countries. Furthermore, data are not always available from countries for the same time periods. The interpretation of these comparative data should therefore be undertaken with caution.[2]

Demography

The proportion of the population aged 65 and over, 75 and over, and 80 and over shows wide variation between countries; the highest proportions in all elderly age groups are in the countries of Western Europe (see Table 12-1). These 1980 estimates showed Sweden to have the highest proportion of population in all elderly age groups, with 16 percent of the total population aged 65 and over compared with less than 9 percent in Canada and Japan. By the beginning of the next century, the proportions of elderly in the United States and Canada are projected to be similar to those of Western Europe in 1960. In all the Western European countries the proportion of very elderly persons in the population is projected to continue to increase, with Sweden having 8 percent of its population aged 75 and over in 2000.[13]

The continuing decline in mortality rates for elderly populations since the late 1970's has led to upward revisions since this table was prepared. For instance, it is now projected that 13 percent of the population of the United States will be aged 65 and over in 2000 (see Table 1-1). Japan is still the country projected to show the most dramatic increase in its elderly population by the year 2000 but, instead of increasing to 14.5 percent, as shown in Table 12-1, it is now expected to rise to 15.6 percent, an increase of 75 percent in twenty years.[6]

It is of note that Israel, a country with high rates of immigration and a relatively high birth rate, is not projected to show any increase in the proportion of total population aged 65 and over, but the proportion of the Israeli population aged 75 and over is expected to rise, demonstrating the universal phenomenon of increasing life expectancy in the elderly.[12]

Life Expectancy

There is considerable international variation in sex-specific life expectancy at birth, with women having a consistent advantage compared with men (see Table 12-2). Japan, the Scandinavian countries, and Canada all have longer life expectancy at birth than the United States, with Japan showing the greatest average life span for both men and women. For Japanese women life expectancy is only 5.5 years greater than for men— 79.66 years compared with 74.22 years—whereas in the United States women have an advantage of 7.4 years, with a life expectancy of 78.2 years compared with 70.8 for men.

Estimates of life expectancy at birth are affected by mortality rates at younger ages, and it is therefore of interest to make cross-national comparisons of life expectancy for older individuals (see Table 12-3).

Although Japan still has the greatest life expectancy for both men and women reaching age 65, women in the United States and Canada have an expectation of life almost equal to that of Japanese women. Furthermore, life expectancy for both men and women in the Scandinavian and

Table 12-1. Estimates of the percentage of the population aged 65 and over, 75 and over, and 80 and over, selected countries, 1980 and 2000.

Country	1980			2000		
	65 & over	75 & over	80 & over	65 & over	75 & over	80 & over
United States	10.7	3.9	1.9	11.3	4.7	2.2
Australia	9.3	3.2	1.5	10.9	4.3	1.9
Canada	8.9	3.1	1.5	10.4	4.0	1.8
Denmark	14.3	5.5	N/A	14.7	6.7	N/A
France	13.7	5.6	2.7	14.6	5.9	2.7
Germany	15.0	5.5	2.4	15.4	6.0	2.8
Israel	8.3	2.5	1.0	8.0	3.1	1.4
Japan	8.9	3.0	1.3	14.5	5.0	2.3
Netherlands	11.5	4.4	2.1	13.5	5.7	2.8
Norway	14.6	5.7	N/A	14.6	7.1	N/A
Poland	10.0	3.3	1.3	12.1	4.2	1.8
Sweden	16.2	6.2	2.9	16.7	8.0	4.1
United Kingdom	14.9	5.5	2.5	15.3	6.7	3.3

N/A Not available.

Source: United Nations, 1982. Demographic Indicators of Countries: Estimates and Projections as Assessed in 1980. U.N. Pub. ST/ESA/SER.A/82, New York.

Table 12-2. Life expectancy at birth, by sex, selected countries.

Country	Year	Men	Women
United States	1982	70.80	78.20
Canada	1980–82	71.87	78.94
Denmark	1981–82	71.40	77.40
France	1981	70.41	78.47
Germany	1980–82	70.18	76.85
Japan	1982	74.22	79.66
Netherlands	1981	72.70	79.30
Norway	1981–82	72.64	79.47
Sweden	1981	73.05	79.08
United Kingdom	1978–80	70.40	76.60

Source: United Nations Demographic Year Book, 1983. New York, 1985

other European countries is lower at age 65 than in Canada, the United States, and Japan.

A similar pattern is shown for elderly men, although Japanese men at age 65 have a clear advantage over American and Canadian men. By age 75, however, the advantage in life expectancy has changed from Japan to the United States and Canada, which then show longer life expectancy for both sexes than all other countries.

It has been observed that Japanese mortality rates at most ages, including infant mortality, are lower than in the United States. Rates of death

Table 12-3. Life expectancy at ages 65, 75 and 85, by sex, selected countries, 1980–82.

Country	Year	At age 65		At age 75		At age 85	
		Male	Female	Male	Female	Male	Female
United States	1982	14.40	18.80	9.10	11.90	5.20	6.70
Canada	1980–82	14.56	18.80	8.99	11.71	5.13	6.34
Denmark	1981–82	13.80	17.70	8.30	10.70	4.70	5.60
France	1981	13.98	18.17	8.24	10.64	4.41	5.35
Germany	1980–82	13.09	16.77	7.64	9.67	4.34	4.95
Japan	1982	15.18	18.85	8.79	10.75	4.64	5.36
Netherlands	1981	14.00	18.50	8.50	11.10	4.90	5.80
Norway	1981–82	14.36	18.29	8.62	10.87	4.74	5.61
Sweden	1981	14.33	17.99	8.40	10.63	4.45	5.31
United Kingdom	1980–82	13.08	17.18	7.78	10.36	4.67	5.72

Source: United Nations Demographic Year Book, 1983. New York, 1985.

from heart disease are seven to eight times higher for both men and women in the United States at age 50 compared with Japan, and death rates from cancer are higher after age 40 in the United States, particularly from lung cancer. Japan has higher mortality rates from stroke than the United States, and this largely accounts for the differences in mortality at advanced ages.[14]

Factors advanced to account for these differences largely relate to life-style factors such as diet and smoking, which may contribute to lower life expectancy in the United States at younger ages. It has therefore been suggested that behavioral modification in the United States could contribute to the achievement of total life expectancy similar to that of the Japanese.[14] A national program of hypertension control recently introduced in Japan to decrease stroke risk may, however, lead to even greater longevity for the elderly Japanese.[6]

It is of note that the two countries with the longest histories of industrialization, Germany and the United Kingdom, have the shortest life expectancy at birth and at age 65 for both men and women compared with the other countries shown in Tables 12-2 and 12-3.

Economic Characteristics and Health Care Expenditures

The impact of health care expenditures and delivery systems on life expectancy is not known, but in all countries for which data are available there has, since 1960, been an increase in the elderly population and an increase in the proportion of national expenditures for health care, with a higher proportion of those resources being paid for the elderly than for other population groups.[2] Considering the existing international variations in the proportion of elderly persons and the projections of continued population aging, it is of interest to compare some of the economic characteristics of the various countries, the percentage of gross national product being paid for health care, and the changes over time.

For countries shown in Table 12-4 per capita GNP in 1980 varied from a low of approximately $8,500 in the United Kingdom to $13,730 in Sweden, with the United States at $11,500. All countries experienced a marked increase in female labor force participation rates between 1960 and 1980. Economic growth rates decreased substantially for all countries except Norway in the period 1974 to 1981 compared with the previous ten years. The average annual growth rate was lower in the United Kingdom in both periods than in all other countries.[2] The United States was characterized by having much lower overall rates of taxation and social security contributions, expressed as a percentage of GNP, than the other countries.[3]

All the countries for which data are available experienced increases in health expenditures as a proportion of GNP between 1960 and 1980, but the percentage increase showed major variation. Whereas in 1960 health

Table 12-4. Total health expenditures as a percentage of gross national product, public health expenditures as a percentage of gross domestic product, and percentage change 1960-1980, selected countries.

Total health expenditures
as a percentage of GNP

Country	1960*	1970	1980*	Percentage change 1960-80
United States	5.3	7.5	9.5	79
Canada	5.6	7.1	7.4	32
Denmark	N/A	N/A	7.8	-
France	5.0	6.6	8.9	86
Germany	4.4	6.1	9.6	118
Japan	N/A	4.5	6.1	-
Netherlands	3.9	6.3	8.3	133
Norway	3.7	N/A	6.7	81
Sweden	3.5	7.5	9.4	169
United Kingdom	3.8	4.9	5.8	53

	Public health expenditures as a percentage of GDP			Public health expenditures as percentage of total, 1980
	1960*	1980*	Percentage change 1960-80	
United States	1.3	4.0	208	42.1
Canada	2.4	5.6	133	77.8
Denmark	3.6	6.2	72	79.5
France	2.5	6.1	144	76.3
Germany	3.1	6.2	100	77.5
Netherlands	1.4	6.5	364	78.3
Norway	2.8	5.6	214	83.6
Sweden	3.4	8.8	159	91.7
United Kingdom	3.4	5.2	53	91.2

* Or nearest available year.

N/A Not available.

Sources: Social Security Administration, Office of International Activities, Simanis J. (personal communication), and Long-Term Care in Western Europe and Canada: implications for the United States. Special Committee on Aging, United States Senate. U.S. Government Printing Office, Washington, D.C., July 1984.

expenditures represented between 4 and 5.5 percent of GNP for all countries, in 1980 the range was from less than 6 percent in the United Kingdom to nearly 10 percent in Sweden and the United States. The 1980 data also showed that Japan expended a smaller percentage of GNP on health care than all other countries except the United Kingdom.[3]

Canada presents the most interesting comparison with the United States in that since the late 1960's it has introduced universal health insurance and has added to this a program of long-term benefits. In spite of these major expansions in health and long-term care programs, health expenditures were still below 8 percent of GNP in Canada in 1983 compared with 10.8 percent of GNP in the United States (see Table 5-1).[3]

Although total health expenditures showed major increases between 1960 and 1980, in most countries public health care expenditures grew at a more dramatic rate, increasing in the United States by over 200 percent and by similarly high amounts in Canada and most European countries (see Table 12-4). The increase in public health expenditures in the United States was clearly the result of the introduction of Medicare and Medicaid in 1966 but, during this period, many other governments assumed the responsibility for providing access to health care for their total populations.[2,3,5-8] Therefore, even with the growth of the Medicare and Medicaid programs, public health expenditures in 1980 represented a much smaller percentage of total health expenditures in the United States than in Canada and the Western European countries. The percentage ranged from 42 percent in the United States to nearly 80 percent in Canada and Germany to over 90 percent in Sweden and the United Kingdom.

Similarly, public health expenditures represented the lowest proportion of GNP for the United States compared with other industrialized countries, 4 percent compared with nearly 6 percent in Canada and 9 percent in Sweden.

Public Expenditures for the Elderly

Estimates of per capita public health expenditures for the elderly in 1980 ranged from $975 in the United Kingdom to well over $2,000 in the Scandinavian countries (see Table 12-5). It was also estimated that the percentage of public health expenditures devoted to the elderly ranged from 21 percent in Canada to 50 percent in Norway.[2] In the United States the elderly account for approximately 30 percent of public health expenditures but, as shown in Table 12-4, public health expenditures represent a relatively small proportion of total health care expenditures, and the elderly population in the United States is responsible for financing over 55 percent of their health care costs.[2] Although comparative data are not available, it is likely to be much lower in the other countries shown.

Total public expenditures for the elderly include pensions and other allowances as well as health and long-term care financed from public revenues. As might be predicted, the level of spending on public programs for the elderly in Europe is largely related to the wealth of the country.[2]

Total per capita expenditures in 1980 ranged from a low of $4,400 in the United Kingdom to over $12,000 in Sweden (see Table 12-5). The percentage of GNP represented by public expenditures for the elderly

Table 12-5. Total public expenditures on the elderly and as a percentage of gross national product, and total public health expenditures on the elderly, and as a percentage of gross national product, selected countries.

Country	Year	Total per capita public expenditure for the elderly		Public health care expenditures for the elderly	
		Amount*	Percentage of GNP	Amount*	Percentage of GNP
United States [a]	1981	6,366	5.9	1,212	1.1
Canada [b]	1982	6,096	5.4	1,370	1.2
Denmark [d]	1980	8,499	10.1	2,356	2.8
France [d]	1980	7,993	9.8	1,876	2.3
Germany	N/A				
Netherlands [e]	1982	7,861	8.2	1,534	1.6
Norway [d]	1981	5,005	5.7	2,546	2.9
Sweden [d]	1982	12,293	14.5	N/A	
United Kingdom [f]	1980	4,416	7.7	975	1.7

*Amounts in U.S. dollars.

[a] 1981 Final report of the 1981 White House Conference on Aging: Volume 1, A National Policy on Aging, 1981.

[b] 1982 Policy, Planning and Information Branch, Health and Welfare, Canada, Government of Canada, November 1983.

[c] Does not include social services.

[d] 1980 Country Report for the World Assembly on Aging, 1982.

[e] 1982 H.G. De Gier, An Overview of the Dutch System of Long-Term Care of the Elderly and Disabled", paper presented at the Expert Group Meeting on Long-Term Care of the Elderly and Disabled, International Social Security Association, Oslo, June 1983.

[f] 1980 Government Expenditure Plans 1982-83 to 1984-85. Cmnd.8494-11, Her Majesty's Stationery Office, London 1982, and Social Trends-12, Government Statistical Service, HMSO, London, 1982.

Source: Long-Term Care in Western Europe and Canada: Implications for the United States. Special Committee on Aging, United States Senate, U. S. Government Printing Office, July 1984.

ranged from under 6 percent in the United States and Canada to 14.5 percent in Sweden, but it should be noted that Canada has a smaller elderly population than the other countries.

Long-Term Care Provision

The definition of an institutional setting varies from country to country, and this creates difficulties in making international comparisons of institutionalization rates. Some countries, such as the Netherlands, have adopted policies for the development of congregate, sheltered, and other types of housing for the elderly; as noted before, the Scandinavian countries and the United Kingdom have focused on the development of an extensive system of home- and community-based care.

Table 12-6 gives estimates of the proportion of the elderly population in institutions and of those in "group quarters" such as congregate or sheltered housing. Institutionalization rates vary from a high of 7.1 percent in Canada to 3.1 percent in Sweden. In most countries with relatively low rates of institutionalization, including Sweden, the Netherlands, and the United Kingdom, the percentage of elderly in sheltered housing and other forms of accommodation tend to be higher and, although only 4 percent or less of the elderly in these countries are institutionalized, a further 5 to 7 percent are in some form of housing development for the elderly.

In Japan, the country with the most recent history of industrial development and a small proportion of older population in the past, long-term institutionalization of the elderly is virtually unknown, and the acute hospital provides the only source of care outside the family.[3]

Comparative data on the provision of home- and community-based services are inadequate to make international comparisons, but one study estimated that nearly 300 persons per 1,000 elderly in the United Kingdom and 260 per 1,000 elderly in Sweden received home nursing and/or domestic help in 1980.[2] Another study showed that in 1980 there were approximately 127,000 home helps in the United Kingdom serving a client population of over 870,000 cases, of whom 89 percent were aged 65 and over.[15] There are no national data for home care provision under the Medicaid, Title XX, or Title III programs in the United States (see Chapters 8 and 9), but Medicare data for 1980 showed a rate of 35 per 1,000 enrollees receiving home health care.[16]

There is considerable debate in the United States as to whether home- and community-based services can provide a cost-effective alternative to institutional care.[17] Although the evidence is somewhat inconclusive, given the much higher proportion of very aged individuals in the Western European countries, institutionalization rates do appear to be significantly lower than in North America. The commitment to community care in the European countries is, however, based on a number of considerations of which cost is not necessarily the most important.[2,8]

The recent Canadian experience showed that following the introduction of the home care benefit there was a consistent pattern of increased demand for home care that leveled off after three years and did not lead to "runaway use."[5] On the other hand, the availability of home health and other community services did not lead to a reduction in the supply of nursing home beds. The presence of an alternative system of care may, however, make it feasible to restrict the growth of the institutional sector over time.[5]

Table 12-6. Population aged 65 and over in institutions and group living quarters as a percentage of the total population aged 65 and over, selected countries.

Percentage of elderly in:

Country	Year	Institutions	Group quarters	Institutions and group quarters
United States (a)	1980	5.3	0.5	5.8
Canada	1978	* 7.1	1.6	** 8.7
Denmark (b)	1980	5.3	0.9	6.2
France (c)	1980	5.2	1.4	6.6
Germany (d)	1980	3.6	0.9	4.5
Netherlands (e)	1980	4.0	7.1	11.1
Norway (f)	1981	5.1	5.7	10.8
Sweden (g)	1981	3.1	6.1	9.2
United Kingdom (h)	1980	3.9	5.4	9.3

* Based on Schwenger, Cope W. and Gross, M. John, Institutional Care and Institutionalization of the Elderly in Canada, in Victor W. Marshall, Aging in Canada: Social Perspectives, Fitzhenry and Whiteside, Toronto, 1980 (excludes data on Northwest Territories, Yukon, and Quebec), Policy, Planning and Information Branch, Health and Welfare, Canada.

** Based on 1976 Canada Census, and Presentation by Cope W. Schwenger, Final Plenary Session, National Conference on Aging, Ottawa, October 1983, Policy, Planning and Information Branch, Health and Welfare, Canada.

(a) Unpublished data, U.S. Census, 1980.

(b) Social Services for the Elderly, Inger Erdal, and, Institutions for the Elderly: Present State and Development Trends Ernest Andersen, Danish Medical Bulletin, Vol. 29, No. 3, March 1982.

(c) Aging in France, 1982, World Assembly on Aging (group quarters include sheltered housing).

(d) Report on the Situation of the Elderly in the Federal Republic of Germany, May 1982, German Center for Gerontology, World Assembly on Aging.

(e) Netherlands National Report on Aging Policy, July 1982, World Assembly on Aging.'

(f) The Aging in Norway: Humanitarian and Developmental Issues, World Assembly on Aging, 1982 (Not including hospital beds).

(g) Just Another Age, Swedish Report to the World Assembly on Aging, 1982, The National Commission on Aging.

(h) Research in the Long-Term Care of Elderly People in the United Kingdom, Patricia M. C. Winterton, 1 presented at the Expert Group Meeting on Long-Term Care of the Elderly and Disabled, International Social Security Association, Oslo, 20-22 June 1983, and Social Trends 12, Central Statistical Office, Government Statistical Service, Her Majesty's Stationery Office, London, 1983; (Includes long-term care wards in hospitals), and Growing Older, Cmnd. 8173, HMSO, London, March 1981.

Source: Long-Term Care in Western Europe and Canada: Implications for the United States, Special Committee on Aging, United States Senate, U.S. Government Printing Office, July 1984.

Summary

Population aging is a phenomenon that has been occuring throughout the world during this century as mortality rates have declined and life expectancy increased. The Western European countries already have a higher proportion of elderly persons in their populations, including those aged 75 and over and 80 and over than are predicted for the United States and Canada until well into the next century. Life expectancy is greater for women than men in all societies and at all ages; therefore the major growth will be in the number of elderly women, the proportion increasing with advancing age.

Japan, the country with the longest life expectancy in the world, which at the present time relies on the traditional extended family in providing long-term care for the elderly, will experience a 75-percent increase in the proportion of its older population between 1980 and the year 2000.

Increasing rates of morbidity, functional disability, and need for health and other long-term care services are universally associated with aging; in all countries for which data are available a disproportionate share of acute and long-term health care expenditures are on behalf of the elderly.

Since the early 1960's, most industrialized nations have introduced programs providing universal access to health care, the financing and control of which varies from country to country. As a result, there has been a major increase in the proportion of public financing of health care in all countries. Also since the early 1960's, most countries have experienced major increases in health care expenditures expressed as a percentage of GNP although the rate of increase has varied substantially.

In addition to a higher percentage of public funding of health care most industrially advanced nations provide universal access to a range of other publicly financed community and social support programs for their elderly and disabled populations.

The United States is unique in the industrialized countries in having had the highest rate of growth in health care expenditures during the past twenty years and in expending the highest proportion of GNP on health care without providing universal access to acute health or long-term care services. Although there has been a major increase in the proportion of public expenditures for health care since the introduction of the Medicare and Medicaid programs, this still represents a much smaller proportion of total national health care expenditures than in other countries.

The increasing costs of the Medicare and Medicaid programs and concerns with the aging of the United States population have led to attempts to regulate providers and to a search for lower-cost alternatives to the institutional bias of the two programs as well as to substantial cost-shifting to beneficiaries (see Chapter 5).

Although Western European countries, with proportionately higher elderly populations, have been able to provide universal access to a comprehensive range of acute and long-term care services, comparisons are of limited relevance to the United States. The profit motive is almost entirely lacking in the provision of either institutional or home- and community-based services in Europe.[7] There would be no political consensus in the United States for the introduction of a centrally funded, fixed budget national health service as in the United Kingdom nor for the extremely high rates of taxation which are accepted in Sweden in return for a comprehensive range of health and social service programs for the total population.

Although there are major differences in population size and structure, Canada undoubtedly provides the best model for comparison with the United States. Universal health insurance was developed to accommodate to a system of voluntary hospitals and fee-for-service physicians. Long-term care benefits have since been added for nursing home and community-based services provided by a mix of proprietary, voluntary nonprofit, and public agencies. This has been accomplished with increases in health care expenditures far lower than those experienced in the United States but with a higher proportion of public health expenditures and a combination of national and provincial government regulation.

It will be of interest to follow future policy changes and developments with regard to health and social service provision in the Western European countries as the proportion of very aged persons continues to increase and to observe the accommodation of the Japanese economy and society to the growth of its elderly population, but the future development of long-term care services in Canada may be of particular significance for the United States.

REFERENCES

1. Long-Term Care and Social Security: Studies and Research No. 21, International Social Security Association, Geneva, Switzerland, 1984.
2. Long-Term Care in Western Europe and Canada: implications for the United States. Special Committee on Aging, U.S. Senate, Washington, D.C. U.S. Government Printing Office, July, 1984.
3. World Health Systems: lessons for the United States, Report to the Select Committee on Aging, House of Representatives, Washington, D.C. U.S. Government Printing Office, May 1984.
4. Brown E. R. Medicare and Medicaid: the process, value and limits of health care reforms. Journal of Public Health Policy 4: 335–366, 1983
5. Kane R. A. and Kane R. L. The feasibility of universal long-term-care benefits: ideas from Canada. New England Journal of Medicine, 312: 1357–1364, 1985.

6. Ohno Y. Health developments in Japan: determinants, implications and perspectives. World Health Statistics, 38: 176–192, 1985.
7. National Center for Health Services Research, Responses of Canadian physicians to the introduction of universal medical care insurance: the first five years in Quebec. DHEW Publication No. (PHS)80-3229, Public Health Service, Hyattsville, Md. February, 1980.
8. Kane R. L., Kane R. A. Long-term care in six countries: implications for the United States, DHEW Publication No. (NIH)76-1207, Washington, D.C. U.S. Government Printing Office, 1976.
9. Shapiro E., Roos N. P., Kavanagh S. Long-term patients in acute care beds: is there a cure? The Gerontologist 20: 342–349, 1980.
10. Gruenberg L. W., Willemain T. R. Hospital discharge queues in Massachusetts. Medical Care XX: 188–200, 1982.
11. Hendriksen C., Lund E., Stromgard E. Consequences of assessment and intervention among elderly people: a three year randomized controlled trial. British Medical Journal 289: 1522–4, 1984.
12. U.N. Demographic Year Book, (1983), United Nations 1985.
13. Oriol W. E. Aging in all nations. A special report for the United Nations World Assembly on Aging. Vienna, Austria, July 26–August 6, 1982. The National Council on the Aging, Inc., 1982.
14. Manton K. G., Soldo B. J. Dynamics of health changes in the oldest old. Milbank Memorial Fund Quarterly, 63: 2: 206–285, 1985.
15. Dexter M., Harbert W. The Home Help Service. London and New York, Tavistock Publications, 1983.
16. Walso D. R., Lazenby H. C. Demographic characteristics and health care use and expenditures in the United States: 1977–1984. Health Care Financing Review 6: 1–29, 1984.
17. Doty P. Can home and community-based services substitute for nursing home care? Office of Legislation and Policy, Health Care Financing Administration, (working paper), May, 1984.

Index

AAA's, *See* Area Agencies on Aging
Activities of daily living, definition of,
  66. *See also* ADL status;
  Dependency levels; Functional
  disability; Index of ADL
AD. *See* Aid to the Disabled
ADL status
  and functional disability, 66, 68–69, 71,
    73–75
  and home care, 143, 147, 150–52, 155–
    56
  and nursing home care, 71, 123, 126–
    27, 220
Administration on Aging, 187, 191, 215,
    217, 218
Adult day care, 140, 198–99, 207, 217,
    229
Age group differences
  in functional disability, 68–75, 143–49
  in health care expenditures and
    utilization, 89, 93, 96–98, 105, 119,
    121–23, 136, 173, 178–79
  in mortality rates, 4, 55–57, 60–62, 105
Aid to the Disabled, 113, 114
Alzheimer's disease, 65. *See also*
  Psychiatric morbidity
AOA. *See* Administration on Aging
Appalachian Regional Development Act,
    114
Area Agencies on Aging, 142, 187, 190–
    97

"Baby boom," 4
  aging of, 8, 10, 13
Birthrates. *See* Fertility rates
Black population
  functional disability rates, 54, 69–74

growth of, 8–11
income, 39, 41–44
labor force participation, 44, 46
life expectancy, 5, 7–8, 59
marital status, 25–27
mortality rates, 59–62
Blue Cross and Blue Shield, 79, 80,
    105

Chronic diseases, 52–54, 59, 62–66
  and mortality rates, 53, 56–58, 62
Cognitive functioning, loss of. *See*
  Psychiatric morbidity
Copayments for Medicare, 81, 107, 110,
    161

Death rates. *See* Mortality rates
Dementia. *See* Psychiatric morbidity
Department of Agriculture, 114, 190
Dependency levels
  in noninstitutionalized population, 68–
    75, 143–45, 147, 150–52
  in nursing home population, 71, 123,
    126–27, 220
Dependency ratios
  economic, 47–50
  social, 20–22
Diagnosis related groups, 81. *See also*
  Prospective payment
Divorce rates, 26–28
DME. *See* Durable medical equipment
DRG's. *See* Diagnosis related groups
Durable medical equipment, 161

Elderly population
  distribution of, 10–12, 14–17

Elderly population (*continued*)
  growth rates, 6, 9–14
  income of, 37–44
  living arrangements of, 28–32
  migration of, 11–12, 14, 16

Federal Disability Insurance Trust Fund, 35
Federal Housing Administration, 114
Federal Old-Age and Survivors Insurance Trust Fund, 35
Female population
  functional disability in, 54, 69–74
  growth of, 9–10, 12
  income of, 39–42, 44
  labor force participation, 4, 20, 32, 44, 46
  life expectancy, 7–8
  marital status, 21, 24–28
  morbidity rates, 53–54, 62, 64–66
  mortality rates, 56, 58, 60–61
Fertility rates, 3, 4, 14, 20, 21
Food stamps, 36–37, 45
Fries, theories of aging and mortality, 52–53
Functional disability
  age-group differences in, 68–75, 144–49
  in noninstitutionalized elderly, 53–55, 66, 68–76, 143–57
  in nursing home population, 71, 123, 126–27

GNP and health expenditures, 83–86
  international comparisons of, 234–37
Grants for State and Community Programs on Aging. *See* Older Americans Act, Title III

HCFA. *See* Health Care Financing Administration
Health Care Financing Administration, data for
  funding of research and demonstration projects, 82, 215–16, 218–19, 221–24
  home health care, 163
  national health expenditures, 83
  nursing home care, 116
Health maintenance organizations, 81, 218–19
HI. *See* Medicare Hospital Insurance Fund

Hill Burton Act, 79, 113–14
HMO's. *See* Health maintenance organizations
Home and Community-Based Long-Term Care Waiver program (Section 2176), 162, 198, 216, 221–24
Home care
  definition of, 140–41
  informal provision of, 142, 146–57
  international comparisons of, 229–30, 238, 240–41
  need for, 143–51
  private payments for, 151–52, 154–57
  public funding of, 141–42, 152–54, 156–57. *See also* Medicaid program; Medicare program; Older Americans Act, Title III; Title XX of the Social Security Act; Veterans Administration
Home health agencies, 142, 202
  and Medicaid, 161–162.
  and Medicare, 160–62, 166–77,183, *See also* Visiting Nurse Associations
Home health care, 140–43, 150–57. *See also* Medicaid program, home health care; Medicare program, home health benefit
Home management assistance, need for, 147–49
Hospital care financing and use, 79–82, 105–7, 191, 220, 228, 238. *See also* Medicaid program; Medicare program; Prospective payment

IADL status
  and functional disability, 66, 68–69, 71–72
  and home care, 147, 150–52, 156. *See also* Instrumental activities of daily living
ICF's. *See* Intermediate care facilities
ICFMR. *See* Intermediate care facilities for the mentally retarded.
Immigration. *See* Migration
Immigration and Naturalization Service, 5
Income distribution of the elderly, 34, 37–43
Index of ADL, 71, 73, 75, 123, 126–27. *See also* Dependency levels; Functional disability
Index of independence in acitivites of daily living. *See* Index of ADL

Institutionalization of the elderly, factors
    associated with, 19, 25–26, 65, 71,
    73, 119, 121, 156
Institutionalized population, morbidity
    rates of, 59, 65–66. *See also* Nursing
    homes
Instrumental activities of daily living,
    definition of, 66. *See also* IADL
    status
Intermediate care facilities, 82, 115–16,
    123
  Medicaid use and expenditures for,
    123–25, 128, 132–36
  Section 2176 waivers and, 221
Intermediate care facilities for the
    mentally retarded, 100–103, 105
Internal Revenue Service, 35
International comparisons
  of health care financing, 227–28
  of health expenditures, 234–37
  of life expectancy, 231–34
  of long-term care provision, 228–30,
    237–41

Kerr Mills Act, 80, 159. *See also* Medical
    Assistance for the Aged; Old Age
    Assistance program

Labor force participation rates, 34, 44,
    46–47
Life expectancy, 4–8, 58–59
  international comparisons of, 231–34
Living arrangements of the elderly, 28–
    31, 146–52
Long-term care
  community-based projects, 217–19,
    221–24
  insurance, 106
  international comparisons of, 228–30,
    237–41
  state initiatives in, 219–24. *See also*
    Home care; Nursing homes;
    Supplemental Security Income
    program

Male population
  functional disability rates, 54, 69–74,
    147
  growth of, 9, 13
  income of, 39–40, 42
  labor force participation, 44, 46

life expectancy, 7–8, 58
marital status, 21, 23, 25–28, 147, 152
morbidity rates, 53–54, 62, 64–66
mortality rates, 53, 56, 58–61
Marital status, 21, 23–26
  and institutionalization of the elderly,
    19, 26, 119, 121, 123–27
Master Facility Inventory. *See* National
    Master Facility Inventories
Means-tested benefits, 42, 44–45. *See also*
    Medicaid program; Supplemental
    Security Income program
Medicaid program (Title XIX), 34, 36–
    37, 80–82, 109–11
  and adult day care, 198
  and community support services, 184,
    197–202
  competitive bidding, 221
  dual eligibility with Medicare, 82, 105–
    6
  expenditures and utilization, 98–105
  and home care, 141, 142, 146, 148,
    152, 154–56, 198–200
  home health care, 159–60, 161–62,
    179–83
  and national health expenditures, 83
  nursing home care, 115–16, 123–30,
    132–37
  personal care option, 197–99
  research and demonstrations, 82, 215–
    17, 219–24
  and veteran population, 213. *See also*
    Section 2176 waiver program
Medical Assistance for the Aged, 80, 115,
    159
Medicare Hospital Insurance Fund, 35,
    80–81, 93, 105
Medicare program (Title XVIII), 34, 80–
    82, 109–11
  dual eligibility with Medicaid, 82, 105–
    6
  enrollees, 93–94
  enrollees and National Long-Term
    Care Survey, 55, 69–70
  expenditures, 89–93
  and home care, 141, 142, 143, 152,
    154, 156
  home health benefit, 81, 110, 159–79,
    181,183
  hospital costs and utilization, 89–98
  Hospital Insurance (HI), 35, 80–81,
    93–95, 105
  and national health expenditures, 83–
    88

Medicare program (Title XVIII)
  (*continued*)
  nursing home benefit, 115–16, 123–32,
    134, 137
  and out-of-pocket expenditures, 106–9
  Part A, 35, 80–81, 93, 105
  Part B, 81–82, 93, 105–7
  and personal health expenditures, 86–
    89
  and prepaid health care, 81, 219
  and private insurance, 106
  and prospective payment, 98, 191, 219
  Supplementary Medical Insurance
    (SMI), 81–82, 93, 105–7
  waivers for demonstration projects,
    215–17
  and veteran population, 89, 106, 213
Medicare/Medicaid Automated
  Certification system, 116, 128–31,
  163
Medicare/Medicaid dual eligibility, 82,
  105–6
"Medigap." *See* Private health insurance
Mental disorders. *See* Psychiatric
  morbidity
MFI. *See* National Master Facility
  Inventories
Migration, 4–5, 11–12, 14, 16
Morbidity, 52–55, 59, 62–66
MMACS. *See* Medicare/Medicaid
  Automated Certification System
Mortality rates, 4, 20, 52–53
  age group, 55–62
  black-white ratios, 59, 62
  disease-specific rates, 56–59, 62
  male-female ratios, 56, 58

NAAAA. *See* National Association of
  Area Agencies on Aging
National Association of Area Agencies on
  Aging, 191
National Center for Health Services
  Research, 83, 215. *See also* National
  Medical Care Expenditure Survey
National Center for Health Statistics, as
  data source, 5, 20, 55, 83, 116. *See
  also* National Health Interview
  Survey; National Master Facility
  Inventories; National Nursing Home
  Surveys
National Data Base on Aging, 191, 193
National Health Care Expenditures
  Study, 83

National health expenditures, 79, 80, 83–
  86
National Health Insurance Act, Great
  Britain, 227
National Health Interview Survey, 55,
  142, 143, 152
National Institute of Mental Health, 55
National Institutes of Health, 79–80
National Long-Term Care Channeling
  Demonstration Program, 218
National Long-Term Care Survey, 55, 65,
  142, 143, 147, 152
National Master Facility Inventories,
  116–19, 128
National Medical Care Expenditure
  Survey, 143, 152
National Medical Care Utilization and
  Expenditure Survey, 83
National Nursing Home Surveys, 116,
  119, 123
National Vital Statistics System, 5, 20
NCHS. *See* National Center for Health
  Statistics
NCHSR. *See* National Center for Health
  Services Research
NHIS. *See* National Health Interview
  Survey
NLTCS. *See* National Long-Term Care
  Survey
NMCES. *See* National Medical Care
  Expenditure Survey
NMCUES. *See* National Medical Care
  Utilization and Expenditure Survey
NMFI. *See* National Master Facility
  Inventories
NNHS. *See* National Nursing Home
  Surveys
Nursing homes
  bed supply and staffing of, 116–22
  characteristics of residents, 65, 71, 119,
    121–27, 136
  expenditures for, 132, 134–37
  legislation and, 113–16
  and Medicaid, 82, 115–16, 123–30,
    132–37
  and Medicare, 80–81, 115–16, 123–32,
    134, 137
  research and demonstrations, 215–17,
    219, 220
  Veterans Administration and, 205–6,
    208–13. *See also* Intermediate care
    facilities; Skilled nursing facilities;
    Supplemental Security Income
    program

OAA. *See* Old Age Assistance program
OASDI. *See* Old Age Survivors and
  Disability Insurance
Old Age Assistance program, 79, 80, 113–
  15
Old Age Insurance, 34
Old Age Survivors and Disability
  Insurance, 34–35, 37, 47–50
Older Americans Act, Title III, 141–42,
  156, 183, 184, 198, 219
  Grants for State and Community
    Programs on Aging, 187–97, 200–
    202
Older Americans Act, Title IV, 215,
  217
Omnibus Budget Reconciliation Act,
  1981, 82, 162, 185, 216, 221. *See also*
  Section 2176
Omnibus Reconciliation Act, 1980, 160,
  161
Out-of-pocket health expenditures, 106–
  11. *See also* Private payments, for
  health care

Part A of Medicare. *See* Medicare, Part A
Part B of Medicare. *See* Medicare, Part B
Personal care assistance
  Medicaid provisions for, 197–99
  need for, 147–49
Personal health care expenditures, 86–88,
  107–9
Physicians, distribution of, 87
Population
  distribution by state, 10–12, 15, 17
  migration, 4, 11, 16
  projections of elderly, 5–6, 8–14
  projections of total growth, 5–6, 8–
  13
Poverty rates, 39, 41, 42, 44
Private health insurance, 79–80, 86–87,
  105–7, 142, 181, 205, 213
Private payments
  for health care, 87, 106–9
  for home care, 142, 152–57
  for nursing home care, 132, 134, 137
Prospective payment
  for home health care, 161–62
  for hospital care, 81, 98, 191
  for long-term care, 219
Psychiatric morbidity, 53, 55, 59, 64–67,
  75–76
Public health expenditures, 83–87, 235–
  37, 240

Racial differences in
  functional disability, 54, 69–74
  income, 39, 41–44
  life expectancy, 7–8, 59
  mortality rates, 59–62

SDAT (Senile Dementia of the Alzheimer
  Type), 65. *See also* Psychiatric
  morbidity
Section 222, Medicare Waivers, 216, 217
Section 232 of the Housing Act, 114
Section 1115, Medicaid Waivers, 216,
  217, 218
Section 2176, Home and Community-
  Based Long-Term Care Waiver
  program, 162, 198, 216, 221–24
S/HMO. *See* Social/Health Maintenance
  Organization
Sickness Insurance Act, Germany, 1883,
  227
Skilled nursing facilities, 81–82, 115–16,
  123–35
  Medicaid and, 124–25, 128–30, 132–
  33, 135
  Medicare and, 123, 128–32
Small Business Administration, 114
SMI. *See* Medicare program,
  Supplementary Medical Insurance
SNF. *See* Skilled nursing facilities
Social/Health Maintenance Organization,
  218–19
Social Security Act, 1935, 34–35, 48, 79,
  80, 113–14, 115. *See also*
  Supplemental Security Income
  program; Medicare program;
  Medicaid program; Title XX of the
  Social Security Act
Social Security Administration
  as data source, 5, 37
  and Supplemental Security Income
  program, 36, 200
Social Security Income, 34–35, 37–39,
  47–50, 81
Social Services Block Grant. *See* Title
  XX of the Social Security Act
SSA. *See* Social Security Administration
SSI. *See* Supplemental Security Income
  program
State Agencies on Aging, 142, 187
State initiatives in long-term care, 219–24
State variation
  in elderly population, 10–12, 14–17
  in health expenditure growth, 87–89

State variation (*continued*)
   in median income, 39, 43
   in Medicaid home health benefit, 179–82
   in Medicaid non-institutional long-term provision, 197–200
   in Medicaid nursing home benefit, 128–30, 132–35
   in Medicaid aged recipients, 98, 104
   in Medicare home health benefits, 163, 166–70
   in Medicare nursing home benefits, 128–32
   in nursing home provision, 117–20, 129–30
   in Supplemental Security Income, 44–45
   in Title XX programs, 185–86, 188–89
   in total population, 15
Supplemental Security Income program, 34–37, 42, 44, 50, 114
   and community-based programs, 186, 196, 220, 221
   and institutional care, 128, 136, 198, 200–201

Tax Equity and Fiscal Responsibility Act, 1982, 115, 220
Title III. *See* Older Americans Act
Title IV. *See* Older Americans Act
Title XVI. *See* Supplemental Security Income program
Title XVIII. *See* Medicare program

Title XIX. *See* Medicaid program
Title XX of the Social Security Act, 141–42, 183, 215, 219
   Social Services Block Grant, 184–89, 197–98, 200–202

U.S. Bureau of the Census, as data source, 5, 20, 37
U.S. Department of Agriculture, 114, 190
U.S. Public Health Service, 79

VA. *See* Veterans Administration
Veterans Administration, 79, 89, 106
   and home care, 141, 204, 206–8, 212
   and hospital care, 205, 208–13
   and nursing home care, 204–6, 208, 210–13
   and population change, 204, 208–9, 213
Visiting Nurse Associations, 159, 166, 171, 172, 174
VNA. *See* Visiting Nurse Associations

White population
   functional disability rates, 54, 69–74
   growth of, 8–10
   income, 39, 41, 43
   labor force participation, 44, 46
   life expectancy, 5, 7–8, 59
   marital status, 21, 25–28
   mortality rates, 58–62